The Ethics of Pregnancy, Abortion and Childbirth

T0133108

The Ethics of Pregnancy, Abortion and Childbirth addresses the unique moral questions raised by pregnancy and its intimate bodily nature. From assisted reproduction to abortion and 'vital conflict' resolution to more everyday concerns of the pregnant woman, this book argues for pregnancy as a close human relationship with the woman as guardian or custodian. Four approaches to pregnancy are explored: 'uni-personal', 'neighborly', 'maternal', and 'spousal'. The author challenges not only the view that there is only one moral subject to consider in pregnancy, but also the idea that the location of the fetus lacks all inherent, unique significance. It is argued that the pregnant woman is not a mere 'neighbor' or helpful stranger to the fetus but is rather already in a real familial relationship bringing real familial rights and obligations. If the status of the fetus is conclusive for at least some moral questions raised by pregnancy, so too are facts about its bodily relationship with, and presence in, the woman who supports it. This lucid, accessible and original book explores fundamental ethical issues in a rich and often neglected area of philosophy in ways of interest also to those from other disciplines.

Dr. Helen Watt is Senior Research Fellow and former Director of the Anscombe Bioethics Centre, Oxford, UK. She is the author of *Life and Death in Healthcare Ethics: A Short Introduction* and the editor of several books, including *Fertility and Gender: Issues in Reproductive and Sexual Ethics*.

Routledge Annals of Bioethics

Series Editors:
Mark J. Cherry
St. Edward's University, USA

Ana Smith Iltis
Saint Louis University, USA

The Ethics of Pregnancy, Abortion and Childbirth

Exploring Moral Choices in Childbearing

Helen Watt

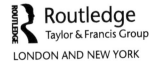

Routledge
Taylor & Francis Group

LONDON AND NEW YORK

First published 2016 by Routledge

2 Park Square, Milton Park, Abingdon, Oxfordshire OX14 4RN
711 Third Avenue, New York, NY 10017

Routledge is an imprint of the Taylor & Francis Group, an informa business

First issued in paperback 2017

Library of Congress Cataloging-in-Publication Data
Names: Watt, Helen, 1962–
Title: The ethics of pregnancy, abortion and childbirth : exploring moral
   choices in childbearing / by Helen Watt.
Description: New York : Routledge, 2016. | Series: Routledge annals of
   bioethics ; 16 | Includes bibliographical references and index.
Identifiers: LCCN 2015035062 | ISBN 9781138188082 (alk. paper)
Subjects: LCSH: Pregnancy—Moral and ethical aspects. | Birth control—
   Moral and ethical aspects. | Human reproduction—Moral and ethical
   aspects. | Bioethics.
Classification: LCC HQ766.15 .W37 2016 | DDC 174.2—dc23
LC record available at http://lccn.loc.gov/2015035062

ISBN: 978-1-138-18808-2 (hbk)
ISBN: 978-0-8153-7193-9 (pbk)

Typeset in Sabon
by Apex CoVantage, LLC

Contents

Acknowledgements

In writing this book, I have been helped by many people, beginning with my family—particularly my father, Ted Watt—and colleagues and governors at the Anscombe Bioethics Centre, particularly David Jones, who made various useful suggestions. I am most grateful to Mark Cherry and Ana Iltis of Routledge Annals of Bioethics and to two anonymous reviewers for significant guidance in improving the text and support with preparing the book for publication. Others who kindly looked at drafts of the manuscript (or parts thereof) include Erika Bachiochi, William Charlton, Christopher Coope, Sally Crippen, Philip E. Devine, Susan Dwyer, Michael Hawking, Claire Hordern, John McLean, Maria MacKinnon, Bertha Alvarez Manninen, Fiorella Nash, Josephine Quintavalle and Celia Wolf-Devine. I thank especially my dear friend Anthony McCarthy for his generous support with the project, his incisive comments on the text, and for so many enlightening and enjoyable conversations on these issues over many years.

Introduction

Pregnancy is a familiar but still in many ways surprising phenomenon, even when it is intended or, at least, strongly welcomed[1] by the pregnant woman. Women delighted by and enjoying their pregnancies may nonetheless be struck by the oddity of the situation: one living body inside another larger body striving to support it—and all this for a whole nine months, as part of the history of every human being![2] It seems an unlikely arrangement, not least at times when the woman experiences some degree of dissonance—minor and temporary as it may be—between her own interests and those of the 'other' she supports.

In terms of naturally occurring close connections (as opposed to more episodic links such as breastfeeding) the closest analogy is perhaps that of conjoined twins. Here, too, there is an enduring physical link between two genetically related living beings who nonetheless retain their own identity. However, there are also striking differences, beginning with the time-limited nature of pregnancy, compared to the conjoined state, which often lasts a lifetime. Pregnancy—as opposed to pregnancy's effects—clearly never lasts a lifetime for the woman, although, like the conjoined state, it can result in harm and even death in some harrowing cases. Significantly, the conjoined state is itself medically a form of pathology, though one that is often positively experienced by conjoined twins themselves.[3] Moreover, some bodily parts are, of course, genuinely shared between conjoined twins, though other parts are not.[4] By contrast, the maternal-fetal link is not a pathology—not, at least, in normal cases.[5] Nor, strictly speaking, are any bodily parts or functions shared between the pregnant woman and the entity she nurtures and encloses.

AIM OF THIS BOOK

In this book, my aim is to explore pregnancy not so much from the physiological—or even the psychological—perspective, but above all from the moral perspective: in terms of rights, duties, risks of various kinds and opportunities to flourish that pregnancy may involve. Abortion is, of course, the context in which these rights, duties, risks and opportunities are often discussed—and inevitably, abortion will also be discussed at some length in these pages. That said, there are other moral issues raised by pregnancy which also call for serious discussion and will be looked at in their turn. Even in regard to abortion, and to the resolution of 'vital conflicts' in high-risk pregnancies, it will be important to consider not merely the moral status of the fetus, but the significance of its location within the pregnant woman and the point, assuming a point can be identified, at which one body ends, and one begins. These considerations are important not only in discussing deliberate infliction of bodily harm but also, I will argue, in discussing deliberate expulsion and/or deliberate invasion of human bodies in ways foreseen, but not intended, to cause such harm.

There are, I maintain, two kinds of mistake we can make in regard to 'pregnancy ethics'. More will be said about these later on: very briefly, one mistake is to treat the bodily location of the fetus in the woman as morally conclusive for the woman's right to act as she wishes in choices that will or may affect the fetus or the child long-term. On this view—a view uncommon in its strongest form—once we know the fetus is within the pregnant woman, we should accept that she is morally free, in every sense, to make such decisions as she wishes, whether in regard to abortion or to the use of alcohol or drugs. Leaving aside the fact that some decisions during pregnancy can affect the child well into adulthood, this approach—so most of us believe—does not do justice to the status of the fetus or to the pregnancy relationship. Most women who are now, or who have been, pregnant, including those who would describe themselves as pro-choice, would reject such a one-dimensional account of their entitlements in pregnancy. They would also reject any suggestion that third parties whose choices may affect the fetus are morally responsible for harm done to the fetus only to the extent that the pregnant woman has opposed or would oppose such harm. (For example, if pollution from a factory is causing miscarriages or other fetal harm, there is no need to wait for the reactions of the women affected—morally significant as these reactions may be—before calling the factory to account.)

However, there is a 'mirror image' to seeing pregnancy as an area where bodily location is in all cases morally conclusive, and this opposite approach involves a different kind of distortion—or so I want to argue. This opposite approach treats pregnancy as no more—though, it is urged, no less—than just another way in which one moral subject (in this case, a pregnant woman) can 'be a neighbor' to a second moral subject. Pregnancy is, on this view, rather like the relationship between a child astronaut and a space capsule under (hopefully responsible) adult control. The womb is seen as something valuable for protecting children, and as such generously offered by the woman, but without this support necessarily carrying any special relational significance—at least where the woman and fetus are not genetically related. Those taking this approach may see the woman who 'rescues' an abandoned frozen embryo as acting as a 'good neighbor' or 'Good Samaritan' to the embryo/fetus without thereby becoming a mother, any more than a woman who breastfeeds an abandoned infant until other carers can take over.[6] Again, this approach does not, I will argue, do justice to the familial aspect of pregnancy or the physical closeness of the bond. A pregnant woman is more than just a *neighbor* to the fetus (a position canvassed in my second chapter on 'The Neighborly Pregnancy'); that is the reason why most women see their own pregnancies as such a serious matter. Nor is the woman's becoming pregnant in the first place, whether sexually or via artificial means, just another way of assuming a neighborly relationship towards some other human being. If the status of the fetus is indeed morally conclusive for some questions raised by pregnancy, so too are facts about its bodily relationship with the woman who gestates. When considering maternal-fetal surgery, for example, that bodily relationship will be very important: it is simply not possible to treat a fetus except 'through' the body of the woman, whose own views on the benefits and burdens of treatments and whose sui generis custodial role will need to be addressed.

What social function does or should pregnancy serve in regard to the pregnant woman and others—beginning with the father? How does pregnancy relate to parenthood (a question discussed in the third chapter on 'The Maternal Pregnancy'), and what might follow in terms of negotiating conflicts or perceived conflicts with the fetus or, indeed, pursuing egg or embryo donation? May pregnancy be delegated to surrogates, or ended if unwanted or unsafe? Are there morally better and worse ways of approaching pregnancy or the possibility of pregnancy, whether one's own or that of another? (This is a question discussed in the final chapter on 'The Spousal Pregnancy', which explores the significance of pregnancy in relation to prior commitments, including marital commitments.)[7] Much remains to think about on questions such as these even after addressing the status of the fetus, an issue addressed in the opening chapter on 'The Uni-Personal Pregnancy', though relevant to other chapters too. Subsequent chapters will explore a range of questions, beginning with abortion but not ending with abortion: questions which our views on fetal status offer only partial help in resolving.

PREGNANCY AND PATHOLOGY

Whatever our approach to the status of the fetus and other aspects of 'pregnancy ethics', there is one point on which there should be unanimity: pregnancy—or at least, normal uterine or pre-uterine pregnancy—is not a disease. Not only is this clear to most of us intuitively, but a closer look at the physiology of pregnancy fully bears out this impression. The womb is, it seems, functionally oriented towards the pregnancy it (or, rather, the pregnant woman) carries, just as the woman's fallopian tube is oriented towards transporting first the sperm to the ovum after intercourse and then the embryo to the womb. Pregnancy is, indeed, a goal-directed *activity*, not a passive state for either woman or embryo.[8] Thus the fallopian tube with its hair-like 'cilia' wafts the embryo towards the womb, which then actively attracts it to landing platforms ('pinopodes'),[9] allowing its own intensely active burrowing-in. Chemical signals are launched from either side, in the interests of securing and guarding implantation: the embryo may well die at any stage, but there are processes which seek to prevent that. After implantation, interaction continues until the end of pregnancy, when signals are directed, not to cementing, but to breaking the bond and producing, all going well, a live birth. Pregnancy is, physiologically, a joint project: it is not—to focus simply on the woman's own bodily functioning—a mere 'fetal imposition', for all the stresses it may bring.

SHARING OF PARTS

Does pregnancy involve a sharing of organs, in the course of all this joint activity? Interestingly, despite the close bodily connection, there is no part or organ which is clearly common to the woman and fetus. The placenta is sometimes cited as such a part; however, the placenta is really composed of two parts, one of fetal origin, the other of maternal origin—the latter, smaller part produced by the lining of the womb. In contrast, the 'fetal placenta' linking what is sometimes called the 'fetus proper' with the woman is produced by the fetus and is normally genetically identical[10] to other fetal parts. This is a genuine organ of the fetus, although one discarded at birth, as its counterpart, the 'maternal placenta', is also discarded.[11] The fetal placenta branches out towards the lining of the womb, and is met by the blood vessels in the maternal placenta that irrigate the space between the fetal 'villi', bringing oxygen and nutrients and removing waste. The blood of the fetus and that of the woman, though allowing these exchanges due to their close neighborhood, remain separate throughout. There is interaction of a more or less harmonious kind, but no obvious sharing of parts.

Many women do, for all that, experience a sense of 'blurred boundaries between self and other'[12] during pregnancy—naturally enough when the fetus is located in a space completely surrounded by the woman's inner (and her outer) bodily borders. Biologically, boundaries can certainly be drawn, though—and more easily than in the case of conjoined twins. This is despite the closeness of the link and even some transfer of cells (maternal cells may be found within the baby after birth and vice-versa). In any event, the woman and fetus share space in a sense, if not actual organs: the womb is 'home' to the fetus it surrounds, while at the same time very much part of the woman who is pregnant. (Such entwinement as a functioning unit is not without parallels elsewhere in human life: breastfeeding and even sexual intercourse involve the functional interaction of living subjects, without either subject losing his or her separate identity.)[13]

DEPENDENCY AND STATUS

One way of approaching 'pregnancy ethics' is to deny—in some cases, firmly—that pregnancy involves a second subject in the *moral* sense (or any *strong* moral sense), whatever the woman's emotional bond with the fetus, and whatever may happen after birth. The fetus may be seen as part of the pregnant woman[14] or, at any rate—if it is said to be a separate individual—as an individual who does not have its own independent moral standing on par with the woman's. This issue is often linked to the dependency of the fetus on the woman—who may therefore, it is said, make all decisions which affect it, since she herself is so closely affected and since the fetus cannot make decisions of its own.

We will be looking at the question of dependency—together with the question of 'custody' of the fetus—at various points in the following pages. At this point, it may be worth noting that, when thinking of dependency relationships after birth, we do not tend to say that dependency *reduces* the moral claim of one individual on another, but if anything the reverse. After all, the dependency of infants—sometimes on a single adult in an isolated area—is not normally thought to reduce their moral claim but, rather, to give that claim some part of its content: if not the part concerned with harm avoidance, which may apply equally to other non-aggressors, at least the claim to positive support, to be factored in with other claims. Similar things can be said about older but profoundly disabled and dependent human beings. 'Viability,' whether of fetuses, newborn babies or adults with life-threatening conditions, is something that varies from country to country, and from situation to situation.[15] Chances of survival routinely depend on technology and/or location: for many, proximity to a hospital; for babies, not being born premature. The pregnant woman's own 'viability' may depend on her getting expert care to deliver her baby, while it would be ludicrous if her moral status[16] were to fluctuate according to the state of the roads or the condition of her transport.

However, there are, of course, many other arguments put forward in favor of a lower moral status for the fetus—arguments which in some, but not all, cases will also apply postnatally to children and some older human beings. We will look briefly in the first chapter at these arguments, which have implications not just for abortion but for other pregnancy issues to be discussed. Questions of unintended harm, whether through medical treatment or through (for example) substance abuse, and questions of transfer of responsibility for the fetus will be examined, in addition to the 'normal' significance of the pregnancy relationship and how this might affect our view of variations on that relationship. Such variations range from surrogacy to ectogenesis and even male or animal gestation. If pregnancy is itself surprising or astonishing—even in its most conventional manifestations[17]—variations on it can be not only surprising but also, in some cases, disturbing. To what extent feelings of moral disturbance may be rationally supported by reflection on the social role that pregnancy plays in more archetypal cases is a question that will recur throughout this book.

NOTES

1   Amy Mullin observes that: "In reflection on their ethical significance, pregnancies tend to be divided into those that are wanted and welcome, in which case ethical issues are not thought to be salient, or else entirely unwanted, and then abortion is presented as the topic of ethical relevance. The ambivalent nature of many women's responses to pregnancy is ignored, as is the contribution women's partners and others in their communities make to whether or not a pregnancy is wanted" (Amy Mullin, *Reconceiving Pregnancy and Childcare: Ethics, Experience, and Reproductive Labour* [New York: Cambridge University Press, 2005], 73).

2   "Having been gestated and having been born are two of the very few experiences common to all human beings. In fact, they may be the only common experiences" (Sheila Lintott, "The Sublimity of Gestating and Giving Birth: Toward a Feminist Conception of the Sublime", in *Philosophical Inquiries into Pregnancy, Childbirth, and Mothering*, eds. Sheila Lintott and Maureen Sander-Staudt [New York: Routledge, 2012], 237). Of course this misses out the case of ex vivo embryos and perhaps, in the future, ex vivo fetuses, if artificial wombs are ever developed.

3   Alice Domurat Dreger, "The Limits of Individuality: Ritual and Sacrifice in the Lives and Medical Treatment of Conjoined Twins", *Studies in History and Philosophy of Biological and Biomedical Sciences* 29.1 (1998): 1–29.

4   With conjoined twins, we have two organisms present, as we have two 'centres of organisation' which overlap in the area they cover. See Helen Watt, "Conjoined Twins: Separation as Lethal Mutilation", in *The Right to Life and the Value of Life*, ed. Jon Yorke (Farnham: Ashgate, 2010), 338. For a contrary view claiming that some conjoined twins involve a single organism, see Jeff McMahan, *The Ethics of Killing: Problems at the Margins of Life* (New York: Oxford University Press, 2002), 35–39.

5   The case of ectopic pregnancy will be discussed in Chapter 3, together with other life-threatening pregnancy situations.

6   For an example of this approach, see Germain Grisez, "Should a Woman Try to Bear Her Dead Sister's Frozen Embryo?" in *The Way of the Lord Jesus, Vol.3: Difficult Moral Questions* (Quincy, IL: Franciscan Press, 1997), 239–244.

7   A 'spousal' approach to pregnancy can be seen in many opponents of embryo donation (also known as embryo 'adoption' or 'rescue'), an issue discussed in the final chapter.

8   Once the woman realizes she is pregnant, her pregnancy can clearly be 'active' in a whole new sense—but even before that point, biologically, she is far from being a mere passive receptacle. We will return to this point in Chapter 2.

9   Alok Sharma and Pratap Kumar, "Understanding Implantation Window, a Crucial Phenomenon", *Journal of Human Reproductive Sciences* 5.1 (2012): 1–2.

10 Like any fetal part, the placenta can sometimes diverge from neighboring fetal parts in its genetic makeup—for example, because it contains material from a now-dead twin sibling.

11 The human body has other temporary parts besides the fetal and maternal placenta—for example, the milk teeth in young children are discarded when they are no longer needed. More generally, we should not expect to find in the fetus—any more than in the early embryo—an exact miniature of an adult shape, such that even the umbilical cord, despite its fetal origin and active role in drawing on maternal support, is seen as extraneous to the fetus.

12 See Mullin, *Reconceiving Pregnancy*, 91; Brooke Schueneman, "Creating Life, Giving Birth, and Learning to Die", in *Philosophical Inquiries into Pregnancy, Childbirth, and Mothering*, eds. Sheila Lintott and Maureen Sander-Staudt (New York: Routledge, 2012), 170; Iris Young, *Throwing Like a Girl and Other Essays in Feminist Philosophy and Social Theory* (Bloomington and Indianapolis: Indiana University Press, 1990),163.

13 As opposed to people's *sense* of their separate identity, which may indeed be blurred in all these situations.

14 There are obvious objections to this position, from the fact that some fetuses are male, while women are female, to the fact that women bond with their fetuses in a way they would not bond with a part of themselves like a kidney (we will return to this point in Chapter 1). Location of an entity inside another entity does not make it part of that entity; thus sperm does not become part of the woman when inside her, nor does the result of the sperm-ovum combination (this result, whatever sex it is, is not part of the man—but neither is it part of the woman).

15 Peter Singer, *Practical Ethics*, third edition (New York: Cambridge University Press, 2011), 127–8. Artificial wombs, when and if they are developed will, indeed, push viability right back to conception; nor will it be plausible to argue that the embryo is really part of the artificial womb (or petri dish, if that is where it is conceived).

16 Of course, specific claims to positive support can be affected by what is practically available: it makes no sense to speak of a right to immediate treatment where such treatment is sadly inaccessible, unless by this we mean that a right was earlier infringed by, e.g., negligent failure on someone's part to make the treatment available.

17 For a lively popular account of 'the surprising science of pregnancy,' see Jena Pincott, *Do Chocolate Lovers Have Sweeter Babies?* (New York: Free Press, 2011).

1   The Uni-Personal Pregnancy

The topic of this book is human pregnancy, not the moral status of the fetus—an issue which forms merely one important part of the wider whole of 'pregnancy ethics'. This wider whole, which includes a range of questions raised by being or becoming pregnant, takes in the woman's bodily connection with the fetus and the moral implications of that connection for the woman and for those about her. These issues will be the subject of later chapters; this opening chapter will examine the status of the fetus—though many will find my exposition frustratingly brief (or, indeed, otherwise frustrating). For only after some exploration, however summary, of the status of one half of the mother-fetus 'dyad', as the bonded pair is sometimes called, can the moral demands of the bond be explored in a bolder and less tentative way. Having come to a conclusion on the status of the fetus, we are then better placed to ask what follows morally from the fact that the bearer of this status is uniquely enclosed within the body of an adult individual.

HUMAN PERSONAL STATUS

The question for this chapter is whether the fetus is, morally speaking, 'one of us'—a human moral subject or, as some would put it, a 'person', though this word has often further connotations. In this chapter, I will use the term 'person' or 'human person' not in the sense of 'self-conscious individual' (for example), but in the rather generic moral sense of 'full human moral subject'. By that I will mean an individual whose welfare and survival have a special moral importance. I will not assume in advance *either* that human persons are the same as (or exist throughout the life of) individual human beings, *or* that anything specific in the way of self-consciousness or past or current experiences is required to have full 'personal' status. I will look at various approaches to the question of what might be required for personal status, including an approach which sees the response of the pregnant woman herself as determinative of the status of her own fetus, more than any characteristics it may have.

One immediate question we can ask about status is: Did we always have our current moral status? Or was this status something we acquired gradually, or at a certain point? Did our status begin when *we* began? A slightly different question, which we will look at first, is: What essentially are 'we'? Are we (for example) our bodies (that is, our 'animated' bodies, not our corpses)? Or perhaps a *part* of our bodies—our brains or some part of our brains? Are we *constituted* by something bodily which precedes us, as a statue is constituted by a lump of bronze which exists before it constitutes a statue? Are we a *phase* in the existence of the human organism, so that 'person' names a stage in the life of that organism, rather like 'parent' or 'adolescent'? Or are we rather something *non*-bodily—for example, minds, or series of experiences?

ARE WE OUR BODIES?

It is common to think that we are our living bodies—not necessarily conceived in very mechanistic terms—though also common to think that we are not. Certainly our thoughts do seem closely embodied: often we consciously experience ourselves simultaneously as thinking, feeling beings and as bodily beings who relate physically to the people and things around us. It is the same being who breathes—consciously and unconsciously—and uses breath to speak, laugh or shout. It is the same being who hears the words of others and comes to understand what they mean. Even religious views which recognize survival after death sometimes speak of a 'resurrection of the body' which returns the disembodied remnant to its 'proper' role of animating some particular body. Whatever we might want to say about the (actual or conceivable) survival of disembodied minds, such entities do seem radically truncated when compared to a whole, bodily human being.

ARE WE OUR EXPERIENCES?

Some of those who may concede the plausibility of a bodily identity for ourselves will nonetheless reply that it is our experiences—in principle, transferrable into other bodies and/or stored in computers—which make up the 'real us'. Reference may be made to, for example, Science Fiction scenarios in which our bodies are emptied of our memories, which are then transferred to another body. Wouldn't we think of ourselves as going where 'our' memories (or quasi-memories) go—rather than remaining 'in' the now-unconscious body with which we began?[1]

However, those defending a human *bodily* identity will point out that—if we keep to Science Fiction—we can imagine 'my' memories being transferred simultaneously to *two* bodies, or (to move a bit closer to reality) we can imagine two people being 'fed' or 'brainwashed' with material from my biography until 'they' believe that they are 'me'. I can't be the same individual as both these people—so why think that I am either?[2] True, each of the individuals after 'receiving' my memories has (unlike the now-unconscious body we began with) experiences ultimately caused by my experiences— but does that make them *me*? Why not see myself as the original, bodily individual who did once experience things (in between sleeping) but has now lost the memory of these experiences and, perhaps, the very ability to experience?

Moreover, we need to ask, more fundamentally, why we have the experiences we do. These experiences appear to be a function—closely coordinated with other functions—of the kind of bodily life we have. That bodily life surely *involves* experiences; it does not simply *cause* them 'from without' for some discrete entity, whether a soul, brain or brain part. In this respect, we are like nonhuman animals: a 'dog subject' is not something separate from a 'dog organism' (whether a single entity or a string of experiences) but an intermittently conscious *bodily* subject whose experiences, like its other activities, are those of the kind of being it is. A dog chases rabbits because dogs are carnivores and rabbits are prey:[3] whatever psychological links there may be between the dog's experiences, these are all experiences of the same dog subject because they are undergone by the same bodily being—the same living whole, or organism, which has needs, tendencies and so on connected with its bodily type. So too with humans: our experiences are very much a function of the specific kind of bodily entity that seems to undergo them. The very same entity prepares for these experiences, sleeps, wakes and integrates itself as an organism throughout. As mentioned above, we have at least the *impression* of unity on a daily basis: we *feel*, at least, as if *we ourselves* have at once a beating heart, the sensations that go with that, and the thoughts that go with both.

Turning to our search for an individual subject who might be the 'carrier' of our moral status, it is hard to see how rights or interests, for example, could be ascribed to, in particular, an experience or series of experiences: how could a thought (or thoughts) have rights of its (their) own? Such an account seems even less attractive than the view that we are persisting, nonphysical beings who merely interact with pre-existing and quite separate living bodies. It appears that we should, at very least, concede that the body is somehow internally involved in the human subject, even if we do not believe that the subject is present throughout the body's life.

Interestingly, there are some strange implications in the sexual/reproductive area if we are not in *any* sense—not even in a partial sense—our own, entire living bodies. If we are not our bodies, then couples do not make love;[4] only the 'animal beings' with which their minds are associated unite sexually. The idea seems ridiculous and demeaning: this is not how loving couples experience what they do. Similarly implausible and demeaning is the idea that a pregnant woman is a mind *using* a separate womb to gestate, in the way that she might use an incubator or some other 'tool' to bring a child to term.[5] Surely a pregnant woman *is* her own, thinking, feeling and (currently) gestating body: her animated body is *her*, not just something her brain or soul makes use of.

OVERLAPPING SUBJECTS OF EXPERIENCE

Another problem for theories which separate the thinking or feeling subject from the bodily organism is that we risk finding ourselves with *two* subjects, filling exactly the same space and using exactly the same bodily parts and capacities to have these experiences. For any living organism of a sentient kind will, if all goes well, first acquire and then exercise the ability to experience. If we ascribe experiences *also* to a separate 'person' (or pre-personal subject) in the case of *human* experiences, then it seems that we have *two* subjects of experience, existing and experiencing simultaneously in the same location and using the same cerebral/bodily equipment: the animal and the (pre-)personal subject. Isn't that one subject too many?[6]

If we carry this confusion over to the case of pregnancy, we risk suggesting that there are two spatially completely overlapping beings, both of a kind to have experiences: a person and that person's 'animal'[7]—the latter carrying an 'animal' fetus who is itself presumably overlapped by a psychological being of some kind, at least in the case of a fetus who is conscious. So: four subjects of experience here, where we would expect to find at most two—assuming there are no twins or triplets in the picture. Again, this seems quite unreal.[8] The living body must be identified more closely with the experiencing subject.

But perhaps the pregnant woman is not exactly her living body (i.e., a living human animal), but is rather *constituted* by her living body, as a statue is constituted by bronze. The problem here is that the living human organism *itself* appears to acquire, as it develops, the ability to experience: not derivatively via some new (pre-)personal subject it comes to constitute, but in its own right—as part of its developmental plan. The organism does not 'borrow' its ability to experience,[9] but, rather, progressively perfects its own capacities to the point where it can have experiences—although these capacities can of course be damaged later on. Why should we think of some totally new entity appearing[10] when the organism acquires, as it does seem to acquire, the ability to experience? And what happens to that new entity when the organism loses the ability, whether temporarily or permanently? We will return to the question of brain damage shortly.

MORAL STATUS AND DESIRES

If a pregnant woman does not *have*, but *is*, in some fairly strong sense, a living body with high-level moral status, when did she acquire this moral status, and how should we think about status generally? (We are, again, referring to the full moral status known as 'personhood,' and not the lower, though quite genuine, status we attribute to, e.g., our pets.)

Some link 'personal' status very closely to a history of thoughts and feelings, perhaps of a highly individual kind associated with a 'personality'. While accepting that the human individual is a *bodily* subject who began many months before birth, they associate the *rights and status* of this bodily individual very closely with his or her desires. Perhaps our rights and status begin sometime after we ourselves begin as living beings. Morality is, we might think, all about adjudicating between 'interests' formed in one way or another by the desires of those involved. Can't we see a hierarchy of status between 'pre-desire' individuals such as embryos, those with primitive desires such as more developed fetuses and infants, and those with increasingly sophisticated desires like older children and their parents?[11]

This may seem like an obvious way of looking at moral status, one which coheres with the importance we attach to some at least of our own desires and projects. In the context of homicide, in particular, the frustration of desires and projects can certainly make some cases of killing morally worse than some other cases—at least from that perspective. To kill me before I finish my great novel is worse in some ways than killing me after I finish my great novel, since in the one case, though not in the other, a morally relevant desire will be frustrated. At least as an aggravating feature of homicide, past desires of the victim can be morally relevant, as can desires of other people. Killing an aimless and friendless, though innocent, person, while still unambiguously murder, does not have the aggravating feature of thwarting the victim's desires and those of friends. Such killing is, nonetheless, quite bad enough and can indeed have other[12] aggravating features: there may be an especially poignant deprivation if one is deprived of the very opportunity to form[13]—much less succeed in—long-term projects, as will be the case with infants, for example.

Even conceding that desires can be linked with genuine interests which can then be thwarted, it is not clear why we should think that the presence of desires or projects is *always* necessary for us to have interests to be thwarted or fulfilled. Certainly, desires do not seem to be *sufficient* for us to have interests in the satisfaction of precisely those desires. For one thing, not all desires are morally good: some not only may, but should, be thwarted—by ourselves and by other people. Spiteful desires are one example; grasping desires are another. We all recognize such desires in ourselves but also feel (at least in our better moments) that these desires and their satisfaction are not in our true best interests and have no claim to be promoted. Insofar as our characters were to change so that we lost such desires and replaced them with more generous and elevated feelings, we would ourselves be better off, even if past desires were thwarted in the process.

Would we be better off simply because *other* past desires, such as the desire to be good people, would then be fulfilled? No, because we also feel that human beings generally have objective interests in *acquiring* the very desire to be good people, even if this means—or rather, *because* it means[14]— some psychological discontinuity with our 'former selves'.[15] For example, if we became corrupted morally to such a degree as to lose all interest in being a better person, this would not mean that we did not still *have* an interest (that is, an objective stake) in being a better person. *Having* an interest in something is one thing; *taking* an interest in it is another. Then again, some depressed people may lose all or most desires apart from self-destructive desires, such as the desire to end their own lives. Don't they nonetheless have objective interests both in living and in getting back the 'will to live'— as well as other good desires? And while survival to this point may not promote past desires in quite the same way as survival of non-depressed people, it may bring something lacking in the latter: grateful surprise at the experience of perhaps undreamt-of benefits of living and projects newly formed.

INTERESTS AND BRAIN DAMAGE

Another example sometimes used in these arguments is that of brain damage followed by amnesia. Wouldn't an individual with serious brain damage have objective interests in *reacquiring* previous good desires—or at least the ability to experience new good desires (and other good mental states)? Of course, this interest might be *unfulfillable* —but is not the interest still *present*? For example, even if no treatment exists, does not the person have an interest in one being developed—or at least a general interest in health? If the treatment is developed, the brain-damaged human being (whether or not she can, in practice, *access* this treatment) retains her interest in health— more specifically, in this case, the recovery of health. She doesn't need a well-functioning brain to have this interest—which is precisely in *getting* a well-functioning brain of a kind possessed by healthy humans of the appropriate age. In the same way, a very young child does not need a developed brain—or, indeed, *any* brain—to have an interest precisely in developing its brain: something objectively beneficial to it. The brain develops both before and after birth, while it can be damaged before, during or after birth, whether mildly or severely. Both fetuses and infants would certainly *appear* to have an interest in developing and protecting their brains,[16] just as brain-damaged adults have an interest in healing theirs.[17] Nor does it seem that moral status or morally significant interests can come and go depending on current brain states of one and the same human organism. If we imagine a surgeon in the process of brain surgery, it would be ludicrous to suggest that the patient's status could fluctuate during the operation, depending on whether the brain's current structure could support the mental life or capacities seen as requisite for 'personhood'. If I were such a patient, could a surgeon really confer personhood on me and withdraw it in this way?

OBJECTIVE INTERESTS AND BODILY KINDS

There are, most of us believe, certain things that are objectively good for us: we can have an interest in them even at times at which we *take* no interest in them. Parents, in particular, are extremely well accustomed to this concept in relation to their children. Every day, in millions of homes, children are told to eat their vegetables (turn off the TV, stop complaining, do their homework . . .) on the basis of just this kind of reasoning.[18] Nor is pregnancy exempt from such thoughts: many pregnant women see themselves as acting in the interests of the fetus during pregnancy—even sometimes in cases in which the fetus has a very serious anomaly and may die at any time.[19] (Of course, the *existence* of an interest is one thing, and what counts as adequate *respect* for that interest is another, a question we will be exploring in later chapters.)

As one writer comments:

> [P]regnant mothers can readily imagine futures in which their fetuses are unloved, unprepared for, and done violence to; and in all such cases, they can recognize a deficiency of goods *for* the fetus, not just for themselves, and act to ensure that their unborn children are *not* deficient in respect of those goods . . . mothers (and fathers) can care for their in-utero fetus in a loving way even when they know that their child is afflicted with a disease that will lead to death shortly before or shortly after birth.[20]

Objective interests point to things that are 'desirable'— i.e., 'reasonable to desire', at least in the abstract, whether or not they always *are* desired. It is reasonable to desire what fulfills us: indeed, it can be argued that value itself is defined by what is reasonable or virtuous to desire.[21] Certain things fulfill us and others like us, and our interests in these things—the ways in which they help constitute our welfare—are very much part of the kind of bodily beings we are. Organisms have interests in their own well-being, including their 'being' per se; that is how they differ from machines, whose 'good functioning' is entirely a matter of human wishes and intentions. *Human* organisms or 'human beings,' in particular, have interests in a far richer range of 'goods' or benefits or aspects of their flourishing than do other animals. Human beings are fulfilled not only by 'life' in some vague sense but by biologically *human* life—and they are more fulfilled the more their life approaches the ideal, not just in terms of physical well-functioning (though that is certainly one dimension)[22] but in terms of moral virtues such as courage and generosity. There are other things, too, that make a life 'better': knowledge, creativity, friendship and other features of our flourishing grouped by some writers under the title 'human goods'. [23]

Do we not all, in practice, grasp the goodness of these things when we reflect on our own experience and on what we want for ourselves and those we love? Most people will agree that such things are good for human beings, in some morally significant sense. While the exact relationship between human flourishing and specific moral norms may be disputed, less controversial is the claim that morality is made up precisely of the need to respect[24] and (where possible) promote the welfare or flourishing of others and ourselves. On this approach to ethics, what we take to be good need not be 'maximised',[25] least of all if this means the targeting of unoffending people to benefit third parties. On the contrary, any moral theory we adopt will need to recognize on this approach the imperative to respect human welfare in individuals before any attempt to promote it in ways consistent with such respect.

HUMAN EQUALITY

One advantage to connecting moral status with interests—and interests with the kind of being we are—is that it identifies one sense, at least, in which human beings are morally *equal*: a view to which many of us would wish to subscribe.[26] We differ in many ways—including moral praiseworthiness, for those of us of an age to start acquiring this. However, we are all the same *kind* of being,[27] who could (in theory) be fulfilled in the same basic ways, and whose fulfillment is always morally important, as the *same* fulfillment in the life of one and the same living being. Of course, many human beings are sadly unlikely to reach this fulfillment any time soon, at least to any marked degree. However, to say that not all human beings are equally *fortunate* is not to denigrate any human being, in any stage or situation. On the contrary, such a comment may be a genuine expression of respect—and perhaps also sympathy where this is appropriate and willingness to help where required.

The 'objective interest' approach is not 'elitist': the brain-damaged person has the same objective interest in health (though one which may be harder to promote) as the strong and healthy adult. In the same way, the young child has morally significant interests in developing, no matter how far along the path of development he or she has gone, and no matter what his or her original endowment[28]—provided the child is a human (and, thus, a rational and so particularly important) kind of being. In contrast, moral theories which say that a human being *acquires* moral status, whether suddenly or slowly, must say that human beings are *not* all equal: some are 'subhuman' or 'semi-human' in status, just as others, perhaps, have 'extra' moral status (for example, more intelligent human beings). The 'better class' of human would be not just more flourishing or fortunate—obviously human beings can vary in that way[29]—but of higher moral importance. That seems unconvincing, even if, once separated out, the 'better class' are seen as equal in moral status at least amongst themselves.[30]

Patrick Lee[31] and others have pointed out the need to avoid reducing moral subjects to mere vessels or vehicles for what is really valuable—such as positive experiences. It is because we care about *subjects* that we care about good or bad futures for those subjects, including ourselves. We also care retrospectively; it is difficult to believe that we ourselves at some earlier, even prenatal, stage were so much less important than our 'elders and betters'—perhaps not even elders[32]—who were already born. Did we not always, by definition, stand to benefit from our own fulfillment as human beings?[33] If so, was this benefit ever really morally insignificant? Again, we should remember that the range of fulfillment appropriate to human beings is incomparably richer than that for other animals we know or, indeed, hope to meet—extraterrestrials aside. [34]

WHEN DOES THE HUMAN INDIVIDUAL BEGIN?

It will by now be clear where this argument is going: if the moral subject is the human organism, and if all human organisms have morally significant interests, the question of moral status will inevitably hinge on when the human organism begins. Assuming for the moment that this line of reasoning holds, we need to ask how early in development we have this human bodily subject. When did the pregnant woman herself begin? and (coming forward some decades) when does the child begin with whom she will be living—sometimes happily, sometimes less so—until they go their separate ways?

What makes one a living human subject? Many claim that it is the potential for *adulthood* that makes the unborn child a human being (that is, a human being 'with potential'), just as the newborn child's potential for adulthood is said to make that child a human being. Pointing to the attributes distinguishing human beings from other animals—a range of special mental powers and creativity—those who take this view will say that young children and embryos have, if not the developed ability, at least the basic capacity for such features and activities.[35]

However, such remarks are misleading if by 'basic capacity' is meant a capacity some human beings or organisms can have while others do not. If what we care about are *objective interests of continuing human subjects*, what we really want to know is when these subjects *exist* so as immediately to have those interests: that objective stake in their own welfare and survival. True, any living being must have *some* relatively[36] 'unblocked' potential to act—if only momentarily—otherwise it (he or she) would already be dead. Life is precisely the tendency of the living entity to act in certain ways in a suitable environment. Having said that, embryos and fetuses can surely be imminently dying—or imminently dying without some major intervention[37]—just like any other organism. While it is true that they still have an 'orientation' to long-term development (perhaps a combination of 'unblocked' short-term and 'blocked' longer-term potential)[38] it may not be true that a given embryo has the *un*blocked potential to grow to be an adult, any more than a given newborn baby.

That said, there are many other tendencies which can reveal the human rational orientation: the organism's *directedness to rationality*, seen in its structure and potential, including blocked potential due to missing or damaged features. Even dying newborn babies show this orientation: for example, anencephalic babies who lack an upper brain will still have vocal cords of a kind that 'ought' to support speech, a lower brain and spinal cord of a kind that 'ought' to support a working higher brain, and genes that 'ought' not only to be present with the others but to have produced this brain many months before. This kind of orientation is found elsewhere in nature; thus kittens are already carnivores before they can eat meat,[39] even if some particular kitten is dying and can never eat meat at any stage, due perhaps to some genetic defect. Or we can think of the biology of sex: a woman's body is oriented towards conception and pregnancy (hence terms such as 'reproductive organs') whatever her actual fertility or reproductive history or intentions. The tendencies inscribed in her body make her a female, a mammal, a vertebrate and—crucially—a rational kind of being, whether she is *currently* rational or unconscious and fighting for her life. Nor are the tendencies inscribed in her body something we can ignore for moral purposes: for one thing, it is impossible to talk about health, disease or medicine without referring to these tendencies.

LIVING WHOLES AND LIVING PARTS

What about the sperm and ovum prior to fertilization—do they not also have a 'potential' or 'orientation' of a kind that makes them living beings? Clearly, both sperm and ovum are alive in *some* sense, just as blood cells are in some sense alive, both when they help to constitute their living source and when they leave that source behind them. However, the life of sperm and ova and blood cells is that of living parts—even if now-separated parts—rather than living wholes. The orientation of sperm and ova relates to future fertilization, not to development as what no gamete can be: a self-organising 'whole' or organism. The very existence of the gametes ends when the sperm and ovum fuse.[40] Robert Joyce comments that "[t]he sperm and ovum are not potential life. They are potential *causes* of individual human life"[41] and points out that there is, in fact, no such thing as a 'fertilized ovum': the sperm and ovum actively engage, at which point they both pass out of existence:

> With the perspective of an evolutionist, who once said that the evolution from non-life to life was a 'leap from zero to everything', we might say that the transition from parent body to offspring is a leap from zero self to all of self.[42]

Only artifacts, such as clocks and spaceships, come into existence part by part, Joyce continues. Living beings "come into existence all at once and then gradually unfold, to themselves and to the world, what they already, but only incipiently, *are*".[43]

One sign of a radical change in orientation, betokening a new self-organising entity,[44] is the chain of events that begins when the membranes of sperm and ovum fuse, allowing the nucleus of the sperm to pass within the membrane of the ovum.[45] While the ovum was oriented precisely to attracting sperm and facilitating their entry, the newly formed embryo is, in contrast, oriented to *blocking* entry of further sperm (or their contents): a sign that we have a new entity with new functions to further or frustrate. While the sperm-blocking function may fail, so that a second sperm enters and damages the embryo, the tendency to block such untoward events is one sign that a new life has begun. If there is orientation to future 'whole' self-organising development (rather than the restricted or chaotic tissue growth that can accompany *failed* fertilization),[46] then we have here a genuine human organism, even in some cases of dual sperm entry.

IDENTICAL TWINNING

But if it is potential of *some* kind that makes an embryo a living (human) organism, what do we say about the potential to give rise to *several* living organisms—identical twins, triplets, etc? Identical twinning from a single zygote (one cell embryo) is one phenomenon often used to argue against the individual nature of the early embryo. (Another is the existence of chimeras, where instead of one original embryo forming two, two fuse into one.)[47]

It may indeed be impossible to *know* in the case of twinning which embryo, if either, is the original individual that budded to create a new embryo and which is the 'budded off' individual created. The problem is not, as some have noted, unique to humans: flatworms, for example, can be divided in two, at which point each half is a living individual. Does that mean that before the split we did not have a single individual? Whether or not we think of the flatworm as surviving in one half (say, the half with the head!),[48] this should not cast doubt on the individuality of the original, 'parent' flatworm.

In some cases, it may be clearer that one particular individual has budded to produce another while surviving the process. Again, this is not unique to natural twinning: any adult could theoretically be cloned if his or her cells were taken and used to produce new human beings.[49] That would not cast doubt on the individuality of the adult, either before or after the process: the adult would simply have given rise to clone 'offspring' in an asexual way. And even if the adult was destroyed in the course of breaking his or her body into clonable cells, that would admittedly end the adult's life, but would not cast doubt on his or her individuality before that point.

Even if some embryos are destroyed in the course of splitting, twinning is the exception that proves the rule with regard to continuous development of the embryo in other cases. For twinning to occur, existing links between cells must be broken down.[50] The orientation of the original embryo is, however, to develop as that embryo, such that it is no accident that identical twinning is a rare event, or that identical twins are at higher risk of being stillborn, or of being born with some anomaly. Note also the difference between the *active* potential of the embryo—its potential *to act* as a living whole, while still alive to do so—and its *passive* potential (liability) to be broken into parts, thus creating one or more new embryos with an active potential to develop of their own.[51]

POTENTIAL AND PREGNANCY

It is, however, essential—and essential to the purpose of this book—to consider the embryo's potential or orientation precisely in relation to the body of a woman who is, or who could be, pregnant. The bodily support of such a woman is vital: literally indispensable for any chance the embryo may have of surviving to infancy or beyond. Indeed, embryos created in in vitro fertilization (IVF) laboratories can only survive a few days in an unfrozen state. An embryo's absolute dependence on a woman's gestational support to develop further has led some to argue that the embryo's potential is itself affected by the choices of others—the pregnant woman and/or IVF patient (and IVF doctor)— even before the embryo is physically harmed. If a woman decides not to continue her pregnancy, or not to begin the pregnancy, in the case of IVF patients, does this not immediately affect whether the embryo has the potential for longer-term development?

It is hard to deny that the right environment is crucial for development actually to take place. However, this is surely true of all our capacities: adults in spaceships, for example, need oxygen to survive. Yet space controllers could not change the *current* potential of astronauts simply by deciding to cut off their oxygen; it would take time for the bad effects to be felt inside the spaceship. Until the astronauts died of lack of oxygen, or were physically harmed, their potential for further biological functioning in the right environment would be untouched by the mere fact that others had decided not to support them.

A woman is not, of course, a remote space controller, much less a subhuman spaceship. To take a more down-to-earth example: the potential of a newborn baby girl is in no way changed by the mere decision of her parents not to feed or raise her (let's say, in a country where women and girls are less valued). True, her potential is oriented to others (her potential to breastfeed, for example, connects with a choice of her mother to breastfeed), but parents who choose not to rear a newborn girl do not by their mere decision change her 'unblocked', actualisable potential—let alone the natural orientation which may involve blocked potential (for example, the child may have a life-threatening, even if treatable, disease). Though perhaps not very different from a baby chimpanzee in her current perceptions, the baby human, unlike the chimpanzee, will be radically deprived if she cannot progress through the appropriate human milestones. Like the embryo and fetus she recently was, such a child is a being of a rational kind, with the orientation, objective interests and moral status that involves. (I have used the term 'rational kind' in preference to 'rational species':[52] theoretically at least, we can imagine members of a rational 'kind' able to interbreed—naturally or via genetic engineering—with members of a non-rational 'kind' from which they were normally geographically separated. Even if this ability made us reluctantly describe members of the two groups as members of the same *species*, the two *kinds* would still be poles apart in terms of their moral status and what counted as their flourishing.)[53]

HUMAN-LOOKING FETUSES (AND EMBRYOS?)

At this point—if not, indeed, before—readers may ask if these conclusions on the status of the embryo and fetus, plausible or not as they may be in some respects, are ultimately credible, given our basic intuitions.[54] After all, if we focus on early embryos, these are not only very small indeed, but they also look and behave very differently from older human beings (including more developed fetuses). They are also much more likely to die than older human beings—or at least, than healthy human beings in developed countries (infants particularly are sadly all too likely to die still in some parts of the world).[55] Granted that women, and men in some cases, can grieve very deeply for a miscarried baby,[56] is it really the same experience to lose an early embryo who is unrecognizable as a human being?

There are several responses to this kind of argument, beginning with noting that women and couples *do* sometimes grieve even for very young embryos (and not only, it seems, for a lost chance of parenthood). IVF couples sometimes bond with eight-cell embryos when they see their photographs: they long for their birth, mourn for their death and have moral qualms about the fate of 'spare' frozen embryos.[57] Then again, a scientist might quibble with the claim that embryos do not look like human beings, pointing out that embryos look *exactly* like human beings (in the sense of human organisms) at that stage of a human being's life. Famously, Robert Edwards, the IVF scientist and embryo researcher, said of Louise Brown, the IVF baby first glimpsed in a petri dish, "She was beautiful then and she is beautiful now".[58]

More fundamentally, though, moral status cannot depend on whether other people—including our own parents—find us attractive or otherwise appealing,[59] or grieve for us when we die. That would leave those of us with serious disfigurements, and perhaps no friends or family who care about our welfare, at a serious disadvantage. Even if a certain emotional response is sometimes 'fitting', there is no reason to expect a perfect fit between moral status and emotional reactions—nor are grief reactions always even called for. As one writer puts it:

> A man might be more upset by the death of his goldfish than by the death of his uncle—he would not necessarily have to reproach himself for that. And of course we should not be drawing earnest conclusions about their respective 'moral statuses'! Nor should we be wondering whether goldfish-days are somehow more valuable than avuncular-days . . . The whole topic invites humbug . . . Sometimes people feel devastated at a miscarriage, sometimes relieved, quite often a bit of both. Each reaction can be appropriate. What dies, however, is the same in either case.[60]

RECOGNIZING MORAL STATUS

Moral status is not, as some argue, 'constructed', whether by individuals or by societies: such a view in fact threatens all of us in making the most basic moral claims of some dependent on the de facto attitudes of others. Moral status is about *recognizing*, not creating, the importance of those whose moral status we identify, in the same way that we expect our own moral status to be, not created, but acknowledged. It would be too easy to say that through our lack of (or attempted withholding of) emotional recognition we could deprive others of their status. For one thing, our emotional response to others is something which does not only change but fluctuates. For that reason, too, the woman's feelings of connection to the fetus cannot be responsible for the moral status of the fetus, psychologically important as these feelings may be. Compare the case of bonding with newborn babies: some women find it easy to bond with their babies (or have already bonded significantly during pregnancy), while other women find it difficult and may be disturbed by their lack of feelings for their newborn. A woman in this situation may be especially disturbed if she feels generally ill-equipped to parent the child: precisely because she has some notion of the gravitas of parenthood, finding herself the mother of someone who radically depends on her, and who will make incalculable moral demands in the future, may be emotionally very difficult. That said, women in this situation will normally be aware that their own lack of bonding and 'readiness for parenthood' does not affect their baby's status: infants no more depend on their mothers (or parents) for their moral status than women depend on their infants (or partners) for theirs. With time, the vast majority of women will bond with their children; before this happens, a child is still a child. Parents do not own their children, whose interests and status are no less important than their own in moral terms, though their ability to further these interests is, of course, incomparably less.[61]

In the words of Sidney Callahan,

> The powerful (including parents) cannot be allowed to want and unwant people at will . . . It's destructive of family life for parents even to think in these categories of wanted and unwanted children. By using the words you set up parents with too much power, including psychological power, over their children. Somehow the child is being measured by the parent's attitudes and being defined by the parent's feelings. We usually want only objects, and wanting them or not implies that we are superior, or at least engage in a one-way relationship, to them.
>
> In the same way, men have "wanted" women through the ages. Often a woman's position was precarious and rested on being wanted by some man. The unwanted woman could be cast off when she was no longer a desirable object. She did not have an intrinsic dignity beyond wanting.[62]

In describing women's varying experiences of pregnancy—and these experiences do vary enormously —we must distinguish between our own 'creation' of flourishing for ourselves and another via a certain role towards that other, and the sheer existence of the other as someone with serious moral claims on us predating such 'creation'. This distinction is often not made clearly—for example, in the following much-cited passage from Hilda Lindemann Nelson:

> Once having conceived, the purposiveness continues: the woman creates a relationship with her fetus. It begins as an act of the woman's imagination, as soon as she knows or suspects she is pregnant. At that point she may be **at odds with her own body** [emphasis added] or she may be in a special harmony with it, as the newly formed fetus both is and is not a part of her own self. If she feels it as an intrusion she may figuratively push it away, distancing herself from it and perhaps aborting it or, after birth, neglecting it or giving it up for adoption. Or she may embrace it lovingly from the beginning, imagining its future and setting it within an existing web of relationships in which it will have a valuable place. Throughout the course of the pregnancy it becomes less and less herself and more and more its own. From the beginning it has a value independent of the meaning-system she weaves around it, but what she weaves also has value—the value of a painting or a song, and not just the value of the honeycomb.[63]

Yes, a pregnant woman can 'weave meaning' around her pregnancy, but weaving meaning around a pregnancy—or better, 'personalising' and building on the profound meaning it already has—is very different from weaving meaning around a nonhuman object which begins with no remotely comparable value, but becomes more pleasing the more we weave. What if the pregnant woman is weaving disvalue rather than value around her baby: does that affect the baby's moral status? Surely not, any more than the woman's unloving partner weaving disvalue around her could affect her moral status, as opposed to her flourishing. A victim of domestic abuse is certainly less flourishing for the fact that her partner hates her and wants to harm her—but morally is in no way less important. Human beings flourish the more they are loved and respected by others—even before they are aware of such love and respect—but inequality of flourishing is something quite different from inequality of moral importance.

Barbara Katz Rothman, another writer who appears to suggest that moral status is conferred by the woman during pregnancy, claims that

> children do not enter the world from outside the world; they do not come from Mars or out of a black box. By the time they are born they have been here, in this world, for nine months: not as children, not as people, but as **parts of their mothers' bodies**. A baby enters the world already in a relationship, a **physical, social, and emotional relationship** [emphasis added] with the woman in whose body it was nurtured.[64]

This statement, while appealing at first sight, seems inconsistent when looked at more closely; nor does it reflect the experience of those pregnant women who *do* love their babies prenatally, whether early or late in pregnancy.[65] A woman who loves her unborn baby does not, in practice, love the baby as a part of herself ("a treasured aspect of her being," as Rothman says later),[66] but rather as a distinct, though intimately connected, individual. In Rothman, as in many others, we see an uneasy coexistence of the insight that pregnancy is a *relationship* (thus Rothman refers to fetuses being in *their mothers'* bodies) and the view that the fetus is somehow still a part of the woman's body. Does a woman have a 'relationship' with her kidney? Is her kidney a "treasured aspect of her being", let alone an "aspect" with which she could have some kind of relationship?

We will be discussing the nature of the pregnant woman's relationship to the fetus, and the precise claims this might involve in different situations, over the course of this book. At this point, it may be worth stressing that human relationships generally are not, after all, just a matter of contingent feelings or untrammelled choice. Indeed, as Celia Wolf-Devine has pointed out, this is an odd thing particularly for a feminist to claim—or to claim in the context of pregnancy:

> [M]aking the existence of a relation between the unborn and the mother a matter of her choice or feelings, seems to run contrary to one of the most central insights of the feminine perspective in moral reasoning—namely, that we already are interconnected with others, and thus have responsibilities to them.[67]

We are not, Wolf-Devine reminds us, atomized individuals, whose relationships are simply a matter of what we choose or how we feel—and that applies to pregnancy no less than to other human interconnections. Any attempt to make sense of the rights, as well as the duties that pregnancy may bring for the woman who is pregnant, and for other people, must take this fact thoroughly on board.

MORAL STATUS: WHAT ARE THE IMPLICATIONS FOR PREGNANCY?

In this chapter, we have looked at theories of personhood, ending with the theory that the fetus is outside the moral circle of 'serious players' until 'invited in' by those already included. Personhood is not, I have argued, conferred by the pregnant woman, or by others, but is rather innate to the living human being or organism. The pregnant woman and her fetus are equally living beings of a specific rational kind. As such, they have significant, objective interests in their own biological welfare and survival, and in other 'goods', including long-term goods, appropriate to the kind of being they are. We are our bodies, whether or not our bodies have a spiritual dimension. A pregnant woman is not a mind using a body, or even a brain using a body. It is she who 'holds' the baby, not some tool—whether the child is right within or just emerging from her.

The maternal-fetal dyad is a linking of two living human bodies and two living human subjects. What that means in terms of integrating the woman's interests with those of the fetus, given that both sets of interests are, I am claiming, of serious moral significance, will be explored in the remainder of this book. The equal moral status of the unborn child, for those who accept it, is only the beginning of the story. Moreover, there is also much in pregnancy to ponder for those still unconvinced of this equal status but who see the life within the pregnant woman as that of, at least, a 'significant other' with whom a relationship has begun.

NOTES

1   See, e.g., Derek Parfit, *Reasons and Persons* (Oxford: Clarendon, 1984).
2   Admittedly, problems of seeming replication could also arise if we accept that a bodily person could be split so that (for example) the upper brain was transferred to a living body missing its own upper brain, while the lower brain continued to organise the original living body. Do I 'go with' the greater part of my body or do I 'go with' my upper brain? Does fusing my upper brain with a second living body create an expanded body for me, or a conjoined-twin style situation? Does it form a new subject, who wrongly believes that she is me?

We could even imagine that the large body left behind was given something to make its brain regrow—and then told all the things that happened to the original individual, even if 'memories' of these things were less convincing to that person than 'memories' seeming to follow the transferred upper brain. It is unclear how much we can learn from such imaginary and (perhaps) impossible scenarios, except for the principle that here, too, one's *conviction* that one is the original person does not necessarily equate to one's *being* the original person.

3　Patrick Lee, *Abortion and Unborn Human Life*, second edition (Washington: Catholic University of America Press, 2010), 42.

4　"Maybe we can say that the couple makes love, but it is their co-located animals that engage in coitus. This view not only sounds absurd (and obscene), but misses the ethically important fact that in sexual intercourse, interpersonal and animal relations come together." Alexander Pruss, "I Was Once a Fetus: That Is Why Abortion Is Wrong", in *Persons, Moral Worth and Embryos*, ed. Stephen Napier (Dordrecht: Springer, 2011), 27. Similar objections arise to theories according to which the person is not a mind but a brain or brain part.

5　See the next chapter for mention of the analogy of the womb as the woman's 'house' or 'property,' an analogy which suggests that the womb is somehow external to her. It would, of course, be possible to take such a view without believing that such 'external' means of nurture could be readily withdrawn (after all, bottles and blankets are external tools used to nurture babies which parents are still routinely morally obliged to use).

6　See Eric T. Olson, *The Human Animal: Personal Identity Without Psychology* (New York: Oxford University Press, 1997), 94–102.

7　It is, however, the case that a powerful impression to this effect can be experienced by female-to-male transsexuals, who report feelings of tension with their bodies when they are pregnant or breastfeeding, which they deal with by seeing themselves as social fathers or fathers-to-be of the child, mysteriously wedded to a pregnant or lactating 'female animal' (Mullin, *Reconceiving Pregnancy and Childcare*, 41–2). Though no one can quarrel with sincere first-hand accounts of how it feels to be in this position, it is nonetheless fair to say that pregnancy is not here given its due as a state of the *person*, not just 'his' or 'her' 'animal'.

8　Alexander Pruss ("Maternal Love and Abortion", http://alexanderpruss. blogspot.co.uk/search/label/abortion) has pointed out the oddity of saying that a woman might love two babies—the infant 'person' who has just appeared and the pre-existing baby that occupies exactly the same space.

9　As seems to be suggested by Lynn Baker: "Your body is a person derivatively, in virtue of constituting you, who are a person nonderivatively. You are a human organism derivatively, in virtue of being constituted by your body that is a human organism nonderivatively". Lynne Rudder Baker, "When Does a Person Begin?" *Social Policy and Philosophy* 22.2 (2005): 28. Baker claims that "a human person comes into existence near birth: what is born is a person constituted by an organism" (p. 36). But she nonetheless admits that it is the *organism* that acquires the properties she sees as constituting the person: "Acquisition of the properties that comprise a rudimentary first-person perspective . . . *by a human organism* [emphasis added] marks the beginning of a new person" (p. 35). And indeed, why should it not be the very same being who develops, in its own right, first the capacity for very simple sensations, then a 'rudimentary first-person perspective' and so on? Why do we need the theory of constitution?

　　Baker is commendably willing to take seriously the biological kind to which human individuals belong. Thus she says that mentally disabled or severely autistic people "are still persons, albeit very impaired, because they have rudimentary first-person perspectives and are *of a kind—human animal—that develops a robust first-person perspective*" (emphasis added). That said, Baker fails to acknowledge the significance of the way that *physiological* features of even the *pre*-sentient fetus mark the fetus as belonging to a kind for whom such a perspective is part of normal healthy development.

10 Thus Jeff McMahan claims that "as it matures, the fetal organism causally gives rise to the existence of the individual who will become a person but it does not thereby cease to exist. Rather, it continues to exist as a mature organism that coexists with the person" (McMahan, *Ethics of Killing*, 305).

11 This position is extremely common. See, e.g., Ronald Dworkin, *Life's Dominion: An Argument About Abortion, Euthanasia, and Individual Freedom* (London: Harper Collins, 1993). For a critique of such approaches, see Christopher Coope, *Worth and Welfare in the Controversy over Abortion* (London: Palgrave Macmillan, 2006). Coope observes:

"It would be quite extraordinary to think of the misfortune that death brings to a three-year-old (perhaps just becoming a 'person'—'a proper little person' its mother might proudly say) as entirely bound up with its little plans and thoughts of the morrow. Even in later life the interruption of 'projects' is quite often trivial. One has had in mind to improve the garden, and has got some way with it. Then one dies, leaving the lawn half cut. We philosophical academics may be somewhat exceptional in this regard—nurturing plans for the writing of articles of indispensable importance to the universe, plans which will come to nothing if the work is interrupted. Death is however a misfortune even for individuals with very modest ambitions. And why need there be any ambitions at all?" (Coope, *Worth and Welfare*, 279).

12 Note that some aggravating features will apply not to the victim's loss or the perpetrator's awareness of that loss but to some other aspect of the relationship between them (for example, a family or other fiduciary relationship). There is still a living candidate to be deprived of something, and in this way there is no real parallel between early death and non-conception in the way sometimes claimed (see, e.g., McMahan, *Ethics of Killing*, 170–1). Homicides can vary not only in their overall wrongness, but in being worse in different ways; it is important to realize this when we think about death in early childhood where 'parental investment' of love and care can be seen as making the death less tragic in *one* sense than, say, stillbirth—at least the child lived long enough for such prolonged love and nurture—but worse in another: some of the parents' actions will perhaps make less sense and be tragically thwarted in some way due to the child's early demise.

13 Arguably there is even *more* reason to acquire personal projects which are then successfully promoted than to promote existing projects, since the acquiring of (worthwhile) projects is in itself valuable: a life containing *both* the acquisition and the promotion of personal projects contains more good things. If that is so, killing me before I start planning my great novel will be a worse harm *overall* than killing me halfway through the writing, though not containing the specific harm of wasting my work on it to date.

14 This is a serious objection to the 'time-relative interests' view propounded by McMahan (*Ethics of Killing*), according to which our interests in our own future are 'discounted' if we will be only weakly related psychologically to our 'future selves'. True, normally we have objective interests in retaining not only our memories but at least the better parts of our personalities, such that any damage to these interests must be recognized alongside any gains in prospect. However, there are certainly cases where there is no discounting of interests (or 'parallel' thwarting of interests) in view of psychological change: the more our personality changes in some areas, the better off we will be—as would be the case with psychopaths, for example. (Psychopaths, like other human beings, have objective interests in basic elements of human well-being such as genuine altruistic friendships and avoiding unjust harm to others. Admittedly, the *achievable* objective interests of psychopaths may be

more modest than those of other people; a psychopath might have a hard-to-promote interest in acquiring a character of deep altruism, but a more achievable interest in more modest, though still worthwhile, goals, such as a mild degree of concern for those around him and/or some degree of protective isolation.)

Note that in the case of fetuses and infants, as opposed to adults, there may be little in the way of existing personality features to lose (and therefore potentially to count against their interest in their adult future). For young children who do have some such personality features, retention of these in the long term may not even be desirable, so that their natural loss in the course of growing up should not be thought to count against the gain of their adult lives. On time-relative interests as applied to fetuses, see Matthew Liao, "Time-Relative Interests and Abortion", *Journal of Moral Philosophy* 4 (2007): 242–56. See also the discussion of McMahan in Frances Kamm, *Bioethical Prescriptions to Create, End, Choose, and Improve Lives* (Oxford and New York: Oxford University Press, 2013), 229–38.

15 A separate point is that one and the same human being can support different 'personalities' and even streams of consciousness; treating schizophrenia is not, however, equivalent to murdering persons.

16 Jeff McMahan, who identifies the subject closely with a part of the brain which is capable of consciousness, denies that an individual who has suffered brain damage which is later treated such that *another* part of the brain enables consciousness would be the same subject as the individual resulting from the treatment. "Even if consciousness can later be generated in the same body (for example, through transplantation of cerebral tissues), **or even in some remnant of the original brain** [emphasis added], the subject of this consciousness will not be the original individual who existed before the destruction of the cerebral hemispheres." *Ethics of Killing*, 441. This seems implausible: if I were to authorize such treatment, knowing that I was about to lose my mental faculties, it seems extraordinary to claim that the post-treatment individual would not be me.

17 Some link moral status to the presence of higher-order mental 'capacities'— i.e., developed powers. However, few would say that these must be instantly accessible (a drunken person may lack them, for example) and once we are prepared to count damaged but recovering capacities, it seems arbitrary to exclude capacities which will take time, development or perhaps even surgery to come to fruition. The same lack of electrical connections may be responsible for lack of consciousness due to immaturity as is responsible for lack of consciousness due to brain damage, or even anesthesia (Patrick Lee, "Substantial Identity, Rational Nature, and the Right to Life", in *Bioethics with Liberty and Justice*, ed. Christopher Tollefsen (Dordrecht: Springer, 2011), 38)— though no doubt with differences too. Is one brain state really so different from the one immediately preceding it that the status of the individual can be so radically improved? Or is having an objective interest in my own future something that somehow gradually 'kicks in' with time, growth or recovery—despite the fact that it is always I myself who will benefit from that future? Neither option seems persuasive.

As Coope notes with regard to the sentience criterion, "the change seems not only to be momentous but miraculous. How could the onset of sensitivity to a pin prick suddenly make the loss of one's future so significant when up to that moment it did not matter in the least? . . . are we to suppose that a wholly new kind of being springs into existence along with the first twinge— or rather, along with the first moment in which a twinge would have been felt if there had been the appropriate cause—the new being, unlike the earlier one, being susceptible to loss" (Coope, *Worth and Welfare*, 203). Compare the plausibility of such a 'miraculous' break with something far better suited as a marker of moral discontinuity: the appearance at fertilization of a new living individual candidate for objective gain or loss—as opposed to the ingredients (sperm and ovum) that combine to form such a candidate.

18 As Laura Garcia points out, "Parents especially do not have the luxury of agnosticism about the human good. Fortunately, one does not need a full-blown moral theory to know that it is good to share toys and bad to bite one's friends. We might look to the goals of parenting, in fact, for clues to the meaning of happiness, since all parents want their children to be happy. In pursuit of this goal, mothers and fathers work to instill such virtues in their children as kindness, honesty, self-discipline, perseverance, courage, loyalty, and the like. They insist that their children eat breakfast, go to school, and do their chores, not because the children want to but because it's good for them" (Laura Garcia, "Authentic Freedom and Equality in Difference", in *Women, Sex, and the Church*, ed. Erika Bachiochi [Boston: Pauline Books & Media, 2010], 29–30).

19 See Appendix.

20 Christopher Tollefsen, "Fetal Interests, Fetal Persons, and Human Goods", in *Persons, Moral Worth, and Embryos*, ed. Stephen Napier (Dordrecht: Springer, 2011), 174.

21 See, for example, J.L.A. Garcia, "The Primacy of the Virtuous", *Philosophia* 20 (1990): 69–91; J.L.A. Garcia, "The Virtues of the Natural Moral Law", in *Natural Law in Contemporary Society*, ed. Holger Zaborowski (Washington: Catholic University of America Press, 2010), 99–140.

22 For an exploration of the good of life and health, in particular, see Helen Watt, "Life and Health: A Value in Itself for Human Beings?" *HEC Forum* (2015), DOI 10.1007/s10730-015-9288-2 (the following sections make some use of material from this paper).

23 The term 'human goods' is often associated with the 'new natural law' approach to ethics taken by Germain Grisez, Joseph Boyle, John Finnis, William May and others (see, for example, Germain Grisez, Joseph Boyle and John Finnis, "Practical Principles, Moral Truth, and Ultimate Ends", *American Journal of Jurisprudence* 32 (1987): 99–151). A belief in the objective flourishing of human beings as something which is and should be central to our moral reasoning is, however, very widely shared.

24 Such respect (or disrespect) also applies to situations in which the person will in any case be deprived of life by third parties: one can murder a person as a member of (say) a firing squad, even if the person will not live any longer if we refrain from involving ourselves causally in his death. More generally, to what extent the wrongful killing deprives us of anything depends on what we are imagining happened instead (for example, death only seconds later, or death a year later, or death 60 years later, and so on).

25 See, e.g., Samuel Scheffler, Consequentialism and Its Critics (Oxford: Oxford University Press, 1988). I address these issues very briefly in *Life and Death in Healthcare Ethics* (London: Routledge, 2000), 11–17). In the present book, I will assume that consequentialist theories recommending (or permitting) the 'maximising' of good, whatever their initial attractions, should be rejected as ultimately unable to do justice to some of our most serious moral intuitions. For a critique of such approaches in a bioethical context, see David S. Oderberg and Jacqueline A. Laing, eds., *Human Lives: Critical Essays on Consequentialist Bioethics* (London: Palgrave Macmillan, 1997).

26 In the words of Christopher Coope, "This conviction about equality in relation to the right to life is indeed something remarkable. It needs to be

correctly described. It is not of course the belief that every murder is equally bad, for any bad action can be exacerbated in all sorts of ways. We should think rather of the claim that in every murder there is, as it were, a core element of equal outrage. This represents a belief very broadly shared. Indeed, we more or less take it for granted. People would think it a mark of civilisation. If someone's 'theory' of the ethics of homicide threatens to endorse inequality in this matter, equality will be dragged in by hook or by crook. When all else fails, stipulation will be called upon" (Coope, *Worth and Welfare*, 166–7).

27 Frances Kamm appeals to the example of a table which can be changed miraculously into a potential person: "Suppose that a table could, by magic, be made capable of turning into a person. The table is not harmed if it is destroyed instead of being allowed to transform." "Embryonic Stem Cell Research: A Moral Defense", *Boston Review*, October/November 2002, http://bostonreview.net/BR27.5/kamm.html (reprinted in Kamm, *Bioethical Prescriptions*, 137–51).

 Coope comments: "Someone who thinks that this is an instructive analogy clearly thinks that the fact that human development is the transformation of a single organism is unimportant when we are seeking to understand the notion of benefit . . . no one would say on [a contrasting] account that we cannot harm a human being while at the toddler stage by depriving it of the possibility of reaching the age of reason. No one would suppose it helpful to talk of a table which might 'reach the age of reason' with the aid of a magic wand. What counts as the good of a being, what is good for it, depends upon what kind of being we have in mind" (Coope, *Worth and Welfare*, 29).

28 We must distinguish between the sheer presence of the orientation and (short-term) potential that makes an individual a living human organism and the differing levels of basic potential which such organisms may have. It is intuitively hard to believe that the feature which gives us moral status should be a matter of degree. Most of us cavil at saying that particularly clever people have higher moral status than less clever people—or that this can be said of those who are genetically 'gifted' but have not yet begun the learning process. It would be small benefit to turn 'elitism of achievement' into 'elitism of basic gifts': what we are looking for is an attribute shared by, and identifying, *all* those of the relevant, morally important kind of being. And once we have identified two subjects as the same kind of being, due to the tendencies and orientation they have, differences in achievement or even underlying levels of potential are easy to accept without sacrificing our commitment to the basic moral equality of human beings. Two people of the same human kind have the same general objective interests; it is just that these interests are—unsurprisingly—unequally fulfilled.

29 Such variations can have their own moral importance, which does not, however, affect the person's moral status; for example, a mildly mentally disabled child might have a greater moral claim than either her more gifted or her less gifted peers to a remedial programme from which she can benefit more than they can. Here the shared objective interest in successful learning has different practical implications for different children.

30 See, e.g., the 'two-tiered' approach argued for by Jeff McMahan *(Ethics of Killing,* 245–65).

31 Lee, *Abortion and Unborn Human Life,* 27. Relevant here are the views of (for example) Peter Singer, who treats disabled babies with conditions like hemophilia as morally 'replaceable'—before or after birth—by babies who would enjoy (even) happier lives (Singer, *Practical Ethics,* 163–7).

32   A full-term fetus in the womb will of course be significantly older and more developed than (say) a 22-week premature baby.

33   This is not to say that interests, and especially pursuable interests, cannot be progressively specified in the course of our lives. For example, my interest in having a happy marriage, if I do marry (and a happy unmarried life if I do not) develops into the interest that my existing marriage be happy. Other interests may be retained but be wrong to satisfy; for example, my life as a polar explorer—which would still genuinely satisfy some if not all my objective interests—may have to go by the board if I have vulnerable dependents.

34   Extraterrestrials, as another form of 'intelligent life', would have (if they existed) comparable moral status to *human* persons: their fulfillment, though no doubt somewhat different, would share crucial elements with our own, as they too would be beings of a rational kind. Alien DNA, like human DNA, and alien physiology, like human physiology, would indicate that aliens and their not-yet-rational offspring had, like us, a rational orientation.

35   As David Boonin rightly observes:
   "Either one insists that all that matters is what the brain can currently do, in which case infants and toddlers will be excluded from the class of individuals with a right to life, or one allows that what the brain will later be able to do also matters, in which case embryos and fetuses will be included in that class from a much earlier stage of development. The challenge is to identify a reason for holding that the potential of the human brain is morally relevant once it has organized electrical activity in its cerebral cortex but is not morally relevant before that point, a reason that is not itself merely an ad hoc device for reaching the conclusion the defender of the cortical criterion wishes to reach" (*A Defense of Abortion* [New York: Cambridge University Press, 2003], 121–22).

36   A frozen but otherwise undamaged embryo has a non-structural and therefore comparatively trivial 'blockage', which nonetheless needs active assistance (replacement by water of the antifreeze it now contains) and not just time to clear. See Jason T. Eberl, "Metaphysical and Moral Status of Cryopreserved Embryos, *Linacre Quarterly* 79.3 (August 2012): 304–315.

37   A patient in the middle of a heart transplant is still alive, even if the transplant is doomed to fail, and even if the patient does not have the inner resources for more than momentary survival.

38   Helen Watt, "Embryos and Pseudoembryos: Parthenotes, Reprogrammed Oocytes and Headless Clones", *Journal of Medical Ethics* 33.9 (September 2007): 554–56.

39   Patrick Lee, "Substantial Identity, Rational Nature, and the Right to Life", in *Bioethics with Liberty and Justice*, ed. Christopher Tollefsen (Dordrecht: Springer, 2011), 36.

40   In contrast, while the embryo, once created, may die at any time, there is no point we can identify in normal human development at which the embryo passes out of existence, to be replaced by an individual of higher status.

41   Robert Joyce, "The Human Zygote Is a Person", in *Abortion: A New Generation of Catholic Responses*, ed. Stephen J. Heaney (Braintree, MA: The Pope John Center, 1992), 33.

42   "It is really a misleading figure of speech to say of the ovum that it is 'fertilized' by the sperm, passively as a farmer's field is fertilized. It is proper rather to speak of the sperm-ovum interaction process. There is no such thing as a 'fertilized ovum'" (Joyce, "The Human Zygote Is a Person," 34–5).

43   Joyce, "The Human Zygote Is a Person", 33–4.

44   An organism is a self-organising whole, which dies when the capacity to organise itself even momentarily is irrevocably lost. This capacity in more developed

human beings is widely linked to the presence of a working brain, although this is increasingly disputed (see, e.g., D. Alan Shewmon, "Brain Death: Can It Be Resuscitated?" Hastings Center Report 39.2 (2009): 18–24). In any event, even if brains are truly necessary to integrate older human beings, that does not mean they are necessary to integrate very immature human beings. The embryo who constructs its own brain is clearly alive before the brain it constructs 'under its own steam,' as it were. As one author puts it, "There is no reason to think that the development of the brain causes the death of that earlier organism, to give way to a distinct organism. Rather, the evidence is that the development of the brain is a stage in the maturation process of the selfsame organism" (Lee, *Abortion and Unborn Human Life*, 82).

45 For a helpful and accessible account of fertilization, see Maureen Condic, "When Does Human Life Begin? A Scientific Perspective", *Westchester Institute White Paper* 1.1 (2008).

46 Watt, "Embryos and Pseudoembryos".

47 Like the problem of twinning, the problem of chimeras, where one embryo fuses with another, is a rather weak argument against the individuality of the early embryo. Just as individual organisms can eat other organisms (normally those of other species), so too—though here as a natural accident—an organism can absorb a sibling organism at the embryonic stage, resulting in its death and the incorporation of its cells into the survivor.

48 Pruss, "I Was Once a Fetus", 24. See also David Oderberg, "Modal Properties, Moral Status, and Identity", *Philosophy and Public Affairs* 26 (1997): 259–98; David DeGrazia, "Moral Status, Human Identity, and Early Embryos: A Critique of the President's Approach", *Journal of Law, Medicine and Ethics* 34.1 (2006): 49–57; Alfonso Gómez-Lobo, "Individuality and Human Beginnings: A Reply to David DeGrazia", *Journal of Law, Medicine and Ethics* 35.3 (2007): 457–62.

49 Cloning from an adult might be done either by 'cell nuclear replacement' (where a cell nucleus from the adult is placed in an ovum deprived of its own nucleus) or alternatively by combining the adult's stem cells with embryonic cells to form a new embryo. In either case, 'building blocks' derived from previously existing human individuals are used to produce an entirely separate human individual. Not all embryos are formed from sperm and ova, as opposed to ova and/or other cells.

50 Lee, *Abortion and Unborn Human Life*, 96.

51 See Helen Watt, "Potential and the Early Human", *Journal of Medical Ethics* 22 (1996): 222–6.

52 For a discussion of species questions, see McMahan, *Ethics of Killing*, 211–17. McMahan, who rejects the use of species membership to mark personhood, nonetheless notes that "the mere fact that membership in the same species is a purely biological relation does not prevent it from being morally significant. After all, even the paradigm of a morally significant special relation—the relation between parent and child—has a purely biological component" (226). This would apply equally to an isolated group of rationally oriented beings which was not coextensive with the wider group of those with whom they could in theory interbreed.

53 We can also imagine a rational kind consisting of just one: for example, mixing human and chimpanzee genes or cells might create a new being of a new rational kind consisting only of itself. Once created, such a personal being would be radically deprived if prevented from fulfilling the rational orientation that its (his or her) body would continue to express—although now in thwarted form. This would be so whatever the individual's potential to interbreed with other kinds of being.

54   It is worth admitting that what we see as credible can be influenced by powerful motives of psychological comfort: "Deciding whether to call an individual a person can affect how comfortable we can continue to be with ourselves and our ways. We don't so much as infer that because an unborn child is not, thank goodness, a person, abortion must be more or less all right. It is, rather, that we need *to keep on saying* that such individuals are not persons—or perhaps not 'full' persons—in order to preserve the freedoms we want." Coope, *Worth and Welfare*, 176.

55   We would not want to say that the children of the well-to-do are more important morally than the children of the destitute, because they are less likely to die naturally. Nor does status neatly track concern to save: our options for saving the lives of some human beings may be limited—for example, after a natural disaster, or in relation to a disease we are unsure how to treat. So too, our efforts to prevent miscarriage may be limited —not least because other good causes are vying for attention —but that is no reflection on the moral importance of the lives that are lost.

56   Anne Maloney comments that:
    "study after study reveals that women who suffer miscarriage report a deep sense of loss and sadness. Many psychotherapists currently recommend that such women hold, if not funerals, then some kind of ritual to honor the life that has been lost and the depth of the pain it causes. Similarly, the most cursory reading of contemporary women's studies literature will reveal a similar pattern emerging with abortion. Even among women who remain putatively pro-abortion, there is a growing recognition of the need to mark an abortion with a ritual, one that allows the woman to acknowledge and grieve for her loss. Loss of what? Loss of what other than her child, and a relationship with that child? Such rituals are emerging all over the West, and Japan even has a name for them, mizugo kuyo" (Anne Maloney, "You Say You Want a Revolution? Pro-Life Philosophy and Feminism," *Life and Learning* 5 [1995]: 36–7).

57   Sheryl de Lacey, "Parent Identity and 'Virtual' Children: Why Patients Discard Rather Than Donate Unused Embryos", *Human Reproduction* 20.6 (2005): 1661–9; Liza Munday, "Souls on Ice: America's Embryo Glut and the Wasted Promise of Stem Cell Research", *Mother Jones Magazine*, July–August 2006, http://motherjones.com/politics/2006/07/souls-ice-americas-embryo-glut-and-wasted-promise-stem-cell-research.

58   Robert Edwards and Patrick Steptoe, *A Matter of Life* (London: Arrow, 1981), cit. Robert P. George and Christopher Tollefsen, *Embryo: A Defense of Human Life* (New York: Doubleday, 2008), 220.

59   That said, recognizably 'human' appearance may be relevant to the question of personal culpability for any wrongful harm to another: "Degree of development at least affects culpability; it is psychologically harder for a woman or her doctor to regard a late fetus as mere tissue; late abortion at least looks very much like infanticide" (Celia Wolf-Devine and Philip E. Devine, "A Communitarian Pro-Life Perspective", in *Abortion: Three Perspectives*, ed. Michael Tooley, Celia Wolf-Devine, Philip E. Devine, Alison M. Jaggar [New York and Oxford: Oxford University Press, 2009], 90). There is also the issue of 'betrayal' of a relationship which has already been at least tentatively accepted (we will return to this in the final chapter in the context of 'fetal reduction').

60   Coope, *Worth and Welfare*, 16–17. Coope would no doubt agree that love for an animal can sometimes be excessive—a mistake. In contrast, it seems wrong to claim that a woman can be mistaken in loving her unborn baby, or that killing her baby against her will is no worse in itself than killing a loved pet.

For an interesting argument to the effect that we can—perhaps surprisingly—draw conclusions from the fact that *some* women love their unborn babies to a judgment on the moral status of unborn children generally, see Alexander Pruss, "Maternal Love and Abortion". As Pruss points out, "the lover also appreciates the beloved as *intrinsically* valuable. Compliments that start with "You make me feel . . . " have a certain inadequate shallowness to them. In genuine love, the beloved is loved for her own sake. The value the mother's love posits in her unborn child is also an intrinsic value."

That said, there does appear to be an arbitrary, or at least a perspectival, side to human affection, even where such affection seems quite appropriate to a given role. Coope notes that "if parents are asked why they want their children to flourish they will not think in terms of an inducement at all—that is to say in the usual case. They might conceivably answer 'because we love them', but this just mentions the kind of wanting involved. Love, in this sense, is just that species of caring for which an inducement is not necessary . . . If someone were to love his children 'because they were valuable' we would expect him to love other people's children in the same way, for no one can intelligibly suppose these last to be of less value simply on account of being someone else's" (Coope, *Worth and Welfare*, 153).

61 "Human beings spend much of their lives dependent on others, and without the nurture and education provided by other human beings no one would survive infancy, learn language, or develop to a point where they can become autonomous. The persistence of human society requires that we reproduce and educate our children in our way of life. Even a liberal/individualist society requires the family, or something like it, to raise children in habits of autonomous judgment and respect for people different from oneself. The family is also the place where people learn the equally important virtue of willingness to subordinate one's own personal interests to the needs of the less fortunate and to the common good" (Wolf-Devine and Devine, "A Communitarian Pro-Life Perspective", 74–5).

Some older human beings will, of course, be incapable of exercising such virtues, and perhaps even of promoting their own interests consciously and responding to their carers. Such people are no less human subjects, with objective interests in respectful care; they are also able to benefit others, not least by eliciting such care from them. As Alexander Pruss points out in relation to loving a spouse with Alzheimer's, to suggest that love which ought to be unconditional should not persist when the loved one acquires such a mental disability is a *reductio ad absurdum* of views restricting 'personhood' to those with certain current mental capacities. Alexander Pruss, *One Body: An Essay on Christian Sexual Ethics* (Notre Dame, IL: Notre Dame Studies in Ethics and Culture, 2012), 39–40.

62 Sidney Callahan, "Talk of 'Wanted Child' Makes for Doll Objects", *National Catholic Reporter* (3 December 1971): 7, cit. Francis J. Beckwith, *Defending Life: A Moral and Legal Case Against Abortion Choice* (Cambridge: Cambridge University Press, 2007), 100.

63 Hilde Lindemann Nelson, "The Architect and the Bee: Some Reflections on Postmortem Pregnancy", *Bioethics* 8.3 (1994): 263. See also below (notes 149, 172 and 192).

64 Barbara Katz Rothman, *Recreating Motherhood: Ideology and Technology in a Patriarchal Society* (New York and London: W.W. Norton & Co., 1989), 91. Of course, even older children can be described *metaphorically* as part of their parents, if by that we mean that parents have a special stake in the welfare of children who 'embody' those who brought them into being.

65 Such love is not necessarily linked to 'planned' pregnancies, but can be immediate and heartfelt in pregnancies that are quite unplanned. See the blog post
of 'Katie Walsh': "I have three baby's (11, 4 & 10 mths) and each pregnancy
that love from the day I found out I was expecting my unexpected ones is
what got me through the morning sickness and cramps and contractions.
I never thought of them as tissue they were babies. The thrill of first heart
beats, u/s and kicks. Feeling hiccups was the best part of being pregnant.
Knowing that their was a little person waiting to come out and meet me and
be held warm and safe in my arms: D Enjoy growing your little bundle of
joy pregnancy is one of the greatest miracles in life." http://www.lifesitenews.
com/news/reflections-of-a-pregnant-pro-lifer?utm_source=LifeSiteNews.
com+Daily+Newsletter&utm_campaign=c5c3d3d4c7-LifeSiteNews_com_
Intl_Headlines_04_19_2012&utm_medium=email

66 Rothman, *Recreating Motherhood*, 161.

67 Celia Wolf-Devine, "Abortion and the 'Feminine Voice'", *Public Affairs
Quarterly* 3.3 (1989): 81–97, available online at http://celiawolfdevine.
com/pdf/Abortion-and-the-Feminine-Voice.pdf, at 10 (see also Celia Wolf-
Devine, "Postscript to Abortion and the 'Feminine Voice'" 1993. The Gutting of the Ethics of Care by Carol Gilligan and Nel Noddings", also at www.
celiawolfdevine.com).

In another paper, co-authored with Philip E. Devine, Celia Wolf-Devine
comments:

"Some feminists have suggested that the relevant cut-off point is when the
pregnant woman begins to bond with the unborn, or feels that a relationship
has been established. She thus confers personhood on it. This view is open to
several objections. Why only the mother? Why can not the father, the state,
or potential adoptive parents confer personhood on it? Furthermore, if personhood is something conferred by others, on what grounds can we object
to members of a tribe who regard members of other tribes as nonpersons or
to Nazis who choose not to confer personhood on Jews?" (Wolf-Devine and
Devine, "A Communitarian Pro-Life Perspective", 89).

2 The Neighborly Pregnancy

As argued in the Introduction, there are two dangers in trying to make moral sense of pregnancy. One danger is that of downplaying the moral and biological distinctness of the fetus, seeing pregnancy as a mere 'condition' of a woman, who alone is the subject whose interests must be considered in choices affecting her pregnant state (at least if no subsequently born child is affected). I have tried to give some reasons in the last chapter for rejecting such a view. Birth is a change of location,[1] not a change of identity, and there are grounds for thinking that a second human subject with morally significant interests is present throughout pregnancy and during, as well as after, birth.[2]

The second danger—the mirror image of the first—is that of downplaying the significance of the baby's location, as if it were a free-floating subject in some non-personal, subhuman environment. In reality, the woman's body is linked to that of the fetus in a way that has irreducible moral importance. Thus when the woman's body is invaded to reach the fetus, whether this is done to harm or assist the child, this invasion has its own moral content, which is absent in most other cases of harming or assisting. We need to take seriously the fact that the woman and fetus are linked in a particularly intimate[3] way when addressing the moral demands of their relationship, and how their bodily involvement factors into these.

It needs to be stressed that decisions which end a pregnancy, whether deliberately or a side-effect of other action, cannot be simply a matter of weighing harms for the woman against harms for the baby. If such weighing was all that was required, resolving these questions might be more straightforward, always assuming that the two parties are morally equal and the *way* death occurs is set aside. Harms to the woman posed by pregnancy and childbirth, if that is the comparison, will rarely approach the seriousness and irreversibility of death for the unborn child. After all, few adults would choose an option that would end our *own* lives in preference to the burdens of pregnancy, and the stresses and sacrifices (though also the joys) of bringing up a child. Even the sorrow of giving up a child for adoption[4] does not seem comparable to death in terms of harm: if offered a choice between adoption and a firing squad, most of us would have few hesitations. Such harm as these options involve or include is, most of us believe, less than death: something that becomes embarrassingly, even painfully, clear when we imagine ourselves and not the fetus literally dying to avoid them.

WHAT KIND OF NEIGHBOR?

However—and this is the topic of this chapter—that fact alone does not solve the question of what a pregnant woman might be said to owe the 'other' she supports. Perhaps the most famous article ever written on the subject of pregnancy—here, as so often, considered in the context of abortion— is that of Judith Jarvis Thomson, first published in 1971.[5] Thomson, a defender of abortion, grants for the sake of argument that the fetus has equal moral status to the woman's, though she herself does not believe that the fetus has this status from conception. Nonetheless, she argues that if the fetus *does* have equal moral status—indeed, a right to life —the question remains exactly what that child is owed by its no less personal supporter.

Thomson gives the example, now known to generations of students of philosophy, of someone who is kidnapped and wakes in a hospital bed to find herself linked by the kidneys to a famous violinist, who is himself unconscious. Nine months of support, if she stays connected, will save the violinist and restore him to health; alternatively, the supporter can unplug herself immediately, at the cost of the violinist's death. Taking her cue from the biblical story of the 'Good Samaritan' who rescues a crime victim lying by the roadside, Thomson argues that we are not morally required to be 'Splendid Samaritans', as opposed to 'Minimally Decent Samaritans', to strange violinists who need our help. Even if a Splendid Samaritan might choose to sacrifice nine months of liberty and remain connected, a Minimally Decent Samaritan could decide to put her own life first and unplug herself from the violinist (or, in the case of pregnancy, the unborn child). In fact, Thomson believes that it could be 'morally indecent' to separate oneself if only a short amount of time is needed to save the other person; nonetheless, one has, she thinks, a right to do this, as no other person has a right to use one's body. While Thomson begins by comparing the violinist case to that of pregnancy due to rape (a situation we will look at in the next chapter), she then extends the comparison to the very much more common case of contraceptive failure.

This is an interesting example, which, for all the criticism it has attracted, often rightly, down the years[6] brings up some very important issues. It is, in fact, more plausible than some other analogies for pregnancy—including some in Thomson's own paper—as it deals with a case in which one is *already providing* support via a connection that would need to be actively severed for one to stop supporting. We are looking, not at the stage *before* the person's co-option to support the violinist, when her bodily integrity has not yet been impinged on, but at the stage when the person is already linked and providing the support. This brings the violinist case a little closer to the case of existing pregnancy, and further away from the case of being asked to donate an organ in the future, or even to gestate an unborn child (say, an IVF embryo) whom one is not yet gestating.[7]

BODILY ATTACKS

How might we begin to look at the issues raised by Thomson's analogy? The first thing to note—at the risk of derailing an important discussion on bodily support—is that abortion is *not*, in fact, a mere 'unplugging' but involves (very obviously, for some methods of abortion)[8] a deliberate bodily attack on the individual supported. Whatever the abortion method,[9] the doctor's aim, at least, will often be to affect the body of the fetus in ways intended and/or known to be lethal (we will return to this issue shortly). As one early commentator observed, things might look different in the violinist case if the only way of detaching oneself was by killing the violinist first—say by drowning or decapitation.[10] This is sometimes presented as the difference between killing and letting die, where many see killing—active causation of the death of another, especially where that other's body is deliberately targeted—as entirely avoidable and morally far more dubious than letting die, which is often unavoidable and blameless if death is not intended.[11] Causing harm by intentionally invading the body of another seems particularly hard to justify in the case of innocent people whose bodily space we normally think of as inviolable. Such invasions cannot be equated with mere failure to aid, or even active withdrawal of aid (assuming at least that these are not themselves aimed at causing harmful bodily effects). If my own bodily borders must be respected—one reason why it was wrong to connect me to the violinist in the first place—why not those of the innocent human being to whom I am connected? Can I undo the wrong of the bodily invasion which caused our two bodies to be linked together by carrying out a wrongful invasion myself—indeed, a far more harmful invasion[12]—of the body of another innocent person?

But perhaps I am entitled to invade this person's body if my own rights are still being infringed? Thomson gives the example of a burglar who has pushed his way into my house through a window by means of a defect in bars put there precisely to prevent such intrusions. Surely I have not deliberately assumed the role of hostess, simply by leaving my windows open on a hot night—any more than a woman who uses contraception, knowing it may fail, has deliberately assumed the role of gestational mother or gestational 'supporter'.[13] May the burglar be attacked by the householder, simply on the grounds that, as she might say, 'it's my house'? If so, would that also apply to the innocent, though unwanted, person who merely stumbles through her window?[14] Thomson does not go into details here on the counterattack she might allow the outraged householder, but the prospects for the hapless guest do not look good.[15]

RIGHT NOT TO BE A PARENT

Thomson herself appears to believe that a 'threat' of this kind (the violinist, the stumbling-in person, the child conceived from rape or failed contraception) may be killed in the course of 'uncoupling' or removing him or her, though she does not believe that the fetus should be killed if it is still alive on removal. Presumably, Thomson would accept that if an artificial uterus is ever developed, the woman should choose, other things being equal, to have the fetus removed to such a uterus rather than destroyed.

Some disagree[16] and claim that the pregnant woman has a right to expect of the doctor, not only her separation from the fetus, but the non-existence of a child at the end of the procedure. And in fact, in the context of abortion, separation often *does* involve, not just deliberate removal or even deliberate bodily invasion, but deliberate termination of life. With late abortions performed by induced labor there is often a procedure of 'feticide' beforehand, where the fetus is lethally injected in the heart to prevent it being born alive.[17] Whether or not separation from the woman and life termination are distinct procedures, the overall aim of an abortion for both the doctor and the woman will often be not only to avoid the burdens of pregnancy for her but to avoid her *being a parent* of the child who would otherwise be born.[18] The aim may be for her to avoid the trauma of adoption, for example: knowing that there was a genetic child somewhere in the world from whose daily life she was excluded.

However, if (as was argued in the last chapter) the fetus is *already a person*, then the fetus is *already a child*: the child, perhaps, of quite specific people, whether or not they will raise it as their *social* child. It is far from clear that a child may be deliberately killed simply to avoid raising or relinquishing him or her: what would we say about a man who killed an infant on those grounds? Perhaps the man has been 'left holding the baby' in an isolated area and is afraid of having to care for the child long-term. But does that justify infanticide?[19] True, there would *be* no baby there to be killed (or so we can imagine) had the man not helped to conceive one[20]—but why should the role of genetic parent give one powers of life and death over one's genetic child? Bertha Alvarez Manninen[21] makes this point in the context of disputes between IVF couples over the fate of frozen embryos:

> If the embryos were regarded as persons, the right to avoid procreation could not entail their destruction, for . . . the right to avoid procreation expands to *preventing* the existence of persons that are one's progeny but it cannot expand to killing persons that are one's progeny, lest we

accord such a right to the parents of infants, toddlers, children, teenagers, and even adult progeny.[22]

SUPPORT AND VIOLENCE: STRANGERS AND SAMARITANS

We will be looking shortly at the parental relationship in pregnancy and what that relationship might mean for those involved, both in and outside the context of abortion. In fact, the issue of bodily invasion is a different issue from that of bodily support: even if we accept that some forms of support are in principle discretionary, it does not follow that innocent people may have their bodies lethally invaded to terminate such support. Duties to support are, it seems, role-related; it is not just a question of the *kind* of support at issue but of who provides or should provide that support. It is fairly clear that *some* forms of bodily support, like donating a kidney to a stranger, are 'beyond the call of duty', while at least some other forms may be owed morally but cannot be socially enforced. And perhaps there are some supportive measures one should only undertake in the first place—assuming one has a choice—if one stands in a quite specific role towards the intended beneficiary. Thus some argue that pregnancy may not be delegated, any more than sex itself with a marriage partner (we will discuss the questions of surrogacy and embryo 'adoption' or donation in the next two chapters).

In contrast, our duties to avoid harmful bodily invasions are *not* in this way role-related. Such duties not to invade the bodies of innocent non-aggressors are quite generally owed to all such people. I am not a 'splendid' Samaritan for refusing to carry out harm (as opposed to failing to give aid) to the crime victim by the roadside, even if my refusal will or may cost me dearly. Imagine that the muggers demand that I implicate myself in their crime by taking a knife and joining in, failing which they threaten me with the same fate. While admittedly the victim—as opposed to the arbitrary ruling of the muggers—is not here the direct cause of my predicament, would the case be any different if I was trapped under the victim's unconscious body, perhaps supporting it and keeping it warm, and would need to cut my way out through that body to escape? What if this would kill the victim, while remaining trapped would 'merely' put me in hospital for nine months? There might be a natural reason for this outcome; alternatively, there might be an arbitrary social reason: delay in getting help might mean the muggers come back, find me trapped and do me serious harm. Even if harm for the person I cut into does not enter as such into my plans, my intended cutting treats what is in fact another person's living body too much like a mere sub-personal obstruction to my end of getting free.[23] We will return in the next chapter to the issue of bodily invasion and foreseen harms; suffice it here to say that it is particularly difficult to defend such bodily invasion in a case in which my victim, though temporarily unconscious, is in no way doomed to die except as a result of the invasion-separation.

The case just described seems one where 'doing the right thing'—respecting the life and body of another person—may well cost me dearly. Refusal to abort could also cost me dearly,[24] either because of an intrinsic physical problem with the pregnancy or because of the hostile or uncaring response of others to my situation. However serious the problem or immoral the behavior of those who ought to help me, it is not clear why this would entitle me to invade the body of someone who is certainly no less innocent than myself, in a way that ends that person's life. Despite the heavy costs of refraining from violent invasion, which in some sense will free me, such violence seems rather difficult to defend, even if the 'neighbor' killed is thought of as a stranger.

SUPPORT AND VIOLENCE: PARENTS AND CHILDREN

If we bring into the analogy a closer role than that of neighbor (or *mere* neighbor), the same distinction applies between choosing violence (including choosing harm by passive means)[25] and simply choosing not to aid. There is a strong presumption in favor of care for a child to be delivered by his or her parents, especially if the child will otherwise die. We regard this not as 'forced labor'[26] but as part of the covenant between generations: just as we were looked after ourselves,[27] there is a presumption that we look after our dependent family members, at least until their care can be reasonably transferred. Not only is this a crucial part of being a parent, on which the very existence of society depends, but it is arguably a form of 'freeriding' to deny our children the benefit of support that we and all other adults have received from our own parents (at least one parent prenatally) and/or some parental substitute. (Admittedly, this fact may not occur to us when we are considering our duties to our children—but it may be helpful to remind ourselves of what we owe to our own parents when we find the thought of some parental role particularly hard to bear.[28])

However, while parents could plausibly have an absolute obligation[29] to refrain from choosing (especially lethal) violence towards their child, whose 'being' is not at their disposal, they do not have an *absolute* obligation to take steps to ensure their child is supported. A parent who is likely to be tortured to death by the Secret Police if he comes out of hiding and supports his child might be entitled to remain in hiding, even if this means his child will or may die.[30] The same parent would not be entitled to target the child deliberately—shoot the child, say, or deliberately starve it, on police instructions[31]—to avoid being killed himself. That is because such choices, unlike the mere choice not to venture out to offer support, actually *aim* at harmful changes to the child's body, not just at withholding aid. In other words, the child's bodily self is intentionally violated here, whether by act or by omission, in morally illicit ways. We might refrain from judging harshly a parent who so acted in fear of dying horribly himself, but sympathy for anyone so tempted, and justified doubts about our own moral strength, should not lead us to condone what was done.

WOMEN: UNJUSTLY DISADVANTAGED?

But—it might be objected—it is women, not men, who can find themselves the primary supporter of a child in the highly routine case of pregnancy, where perhaps only an invasion of the child's own bodily borders can end, without unreasonable delay, any unwilling service as a 'fetal container'. Is it possible that a woman's duties are so different from a man's, in regard to the level of support she can owe in such a routine situation? Admittedly, both she and the child's father must refrain from choosing abortion, on the view I am advancing—in her case, by not having an abortion; in his, by not urging her to do so.[32] However, the outcome of *not* choosing an abortion will be very much more burdensome for her than for him, especially in the months before birth, but very likely after birth as well.[33] Care for the child when it is born is, in practice, more likely to fall to her, while an adoption is likely to be more painful for her, after months of gestating the baby, than it would be for the father. (We will discuss in the next two chapters the rights and 'positive' obligations for parents which might accompany pregnancy and childbirth; here we are more concerned with the burden of any 'negative' obligation not to attack, physically invade in harmful ways or, perhaps, non-invasively separate the child one is supporting.)

It is hard to deny that pregnancy and childbirth can pose heavy burdens (even if not *only* burdens) for those who undergo them. The woman's physiology, combined with social factors, is what makes her incur these burdens—which has led some to say that they are unfair: a 'natural injustice'.[34] It will never be more than half the human race of whom such things could be expected. And yet, if we have *any* duties to support others, these must to some extent track our physiology, on the principle of 'noblesse oblige'. Most of us think that it is possible to acquire prima facie *positive* obligations simply by being physically in a position to assist a stranger—a crime victim, for example, or a starving infant in our close proximity. As Mary Catherine Sommers writes:

> A 'robust' constitution is certainly a characteristic which is relevant to establishing the obligation to render living-saving assistance through bodily means. What is unclear is why having breasts, milk glands, or a womb are not similarly relevant to the starving newborn's or the developing pre-born's need for life-support.[35]

While this comment may not do justice to the more *parental* features of the pregnancy relationship, to which we will turn shortly, it does highlight the fact that any duty to support,[36] where it does exist, will presuppose an ability to do so, as well as a need that it be done. Do we think it unfair that 'robust' individuals (to use Sommers' term) are often, if not always, expected to care for family members and even strangers in some situations? Have they not benefited themselves in the past from the help of countless other human beings? Admittedly, they may not have benefited directly from the person who now needs their help—though if they *have* benefited directly from that person, there is a further claim of justice. But do we not also feel that those who have benefited from others' care—even if not from the *same* others' care—may well have a responsibility to 'give something back', at least with forms of care that everybody needs? Do not societies depend on just such willingness to support as one has been supported? True, the 'robust' or comparatively robust will often need more support from others when they (or we) give support ourselves.[37] Those around us and/or wider social structures should indeed help all of us to make the best use morally of our strengths and advantages. However, if we focus on a given individual, and his or her responsibilities in a given case, is there any way of avoiding the fact that, here as elsewhere, 'must implies can'?

FUNCTIONAL SUPPORT

It should be noted that breastfeeding and, to a lesser extent, caring for the crime victim involve, like pregnancy, functional bodily activity: activity towards which the human body is already in some sense oriented. In this they differ both from the violinist case and from more familiar cases in which people are pressed to become live organ donors: it is no part of the function of a kidney that it be removed and/or made to support the body of a stranger (albeit in a way that then co-opts the kidney's normal functions).[38] In contrast, it *is* in some sense part of the function of human beings—the generic function that benefits the crime victim—that they lift and carry objects, including human bodies of appropriate size. Those who cannot carry need not help the victim (or not in that way—perhaps they could ring for an ambulance); those who *can* carry the victim (for example, to their car) have at least a prima facie duty to do so, if this will save his life. In any event, they may not themselves *deliberately attack* the victim, whether by act or omission, to preserve their independence and avoid the expectation of help. It is one thing to delay 'getting involved' until the criminals are out of sight, simply to preserve one's own life. It is something quite different to delay getting involved precisely in order that the victim will die and thus make no demands on our resources. Active killing of the victim to avoid such demands would of course be similarly excluded; the aim of making die is sufficient, if not (I will argue in the next chapter) necessary to rule out such bodily assaults.

Lifting the crime victim might be expected more of the average man than of the average woman, though either might be in a position to assist.

How do breastfeeding and gestation—two specifically sex-related forms of bodily support—compare with this scenario? Breastfeeding and gestation, while superficially equivalent, may not be as similar as might at first appear: quite apart from the stronger connection one may have with maternity, breastfeeding normally involves a succession of positive choices of the woman to breastfeed. In contrast, an existing pregnancy will often need no further chosen act from the woman (apart from routine acts like eating and drinking) in order to go to term. The bodily link is so intimate in pregnancy that only birth or serious dysfunction or violence[39] will be able to disentangle the linked parties. The difficulty of childbirth can indeed be seen as a measure of the physical 'tightness' of the bond, at least by that later stage. In contrast, while two bodies also interact directly with breastfeeding, this happens in an intermittent and, in principle, readily substitutable way—even if sometimes a particular child's life may depend on a particular woman's aid.

A crime victim who needs lifting into one's car does not 'belong' in the arms of the lifter, except in the most temporary and contingent sense. Morally speaking, he belongs or may belong there temporarily, given the supporter's normally functioning body;[40] however, that is all that one can say. Does a starving infant 'belong' on the breast of a woman who can breastfeed? *Prima facie* yes, but again, only in a rather temporary and contingent sense, if it is not one's own child but a stranger one is planning to hand over to others (ideally, to the mother) at the first opportunity.[41]

The difference with pregnancy is that arguably a child in one's womb is *always* one's own child: [42] functionally, relationally and perhaps also morally, the fetus belongs in the pregnant woman's womb in a rather strong sense, in that it belongs nowhere else (apart, of course, from the fallopian tube and the birth canal, though only en route to, or away from, the womb). The womb is now, if not indefinitely, the baby's 'natural habitat', as the functional activity of both linked bodies—woman and fetus—would appear to show. This makes Thomson's comparison with a burglar breaking in through one's window—or even an innocent person blundering through it—particularly inept. The embryo does not 'blunder' up the fallopian tube to implant in the womb: it directs itself, and/or is directed by the woman's own body, every step of the way.[43]

To say all this is not to deny that the womb or fallopian tube (or breast) remains entirely part of the woman. Nor is it to conflate[44] the question of maternal function with the question of the baby's *entitlement to benefit from* that function by being gestated or breastfed, although the questions are certainly related. There are many distinctions we might want to make here, from the distinction between *beginning* a pregnancy and *continuing* a pregnancy to the distinction between the function of pregnancy and that of breastfeeding, which involves a series of readily transferred positive acts, and is less closely linked to motherhood. More generally, however, 'function' and 'dysfunction' are certainly relevant to our moral choices, whether those choices concern ourselves alone or any offspring we may have. To deny this is to suggest that respect for others and ourselves should be somehow indifferent to *health*, an important aspect of our flourishing.

PREGNANCY AS A DISEASE

Normal uterine or pre-uterine pregnancy is not an illness but a functional state of the body. Physiologically, the womb is no less 'for' the embryo and fetus than a kangaroo's pouch is 'for' the joey who may ride there. Whatever our account of the woman's obligations—and her functioning body is not irrelevant to these—this much at least should be clear. The difference is, of course, that human mothers can actively embrace, as well as reject, their power to nurture their offspring. To say this is not, however, to concede that embracing or rejecting this power, at a point where the power is already being exercised, are morally equivalent responses to the need of human offspring for support.

Feminist writers have often drawn attention to the common, and concerning, 'medicalisation' of pregnancy—as if a woman were to be regarded as ill from the mere fact she is pregnant. Some have gone further in noting that abortion is routinely and bizarrely offered as 'medical treatment' for a body seen as in some way 'out of control'. One writer goes so far as to say that:

> The demand for abortion rights in the name of control speaks volumes: it says that the patriarchal worldview has been right all along, that bodies, especially women's bodies, are undependable, threatening things that need to be dominated and subdued.[45]

Another agrees:

> By lockstepping the woman with her physician, the [US Supreme Court in Roe v. Wade] was not acknowledging her dignity as a person, but was adjusting to something construed as defective in her nature: her inconvenient tendency to produce unwanted "fetal tissue" as a result of her sexual contact with an "infecting" male . . . Doctors who treat normal, healthy physical conditions as if they were deformed are practicing quackery.[46]

A very different view is held by Anna Smajdor, who vigorously maintains:

> There has been a conceptual failure in medical and social and ethical terms to address the pathological nature of gestation and childbirth and to tackle the health problems it involves from a justice perspective.

Smajdor calls for the development of artificial uteruses to avoid this putative dysfunction, adding:

> Just as it was thought absurd that women should vote or ride horses astride, so it may come to seem absurd that they were chained to the degrading and dangerous processes of pregnancy and childbirth simply because of our inability to get our heads round the possibility of an alternative.[47]

Smajdor's comments, startling as they are, serve a useful function in providing a *reductio ad absurdum* of the view that human (and animal?) pregnancy is a pathological condition. Without in any way downplaying the burdens and dangers that pregnancy can bring in its train, to treat pregnancy *itself* as a disease still seems perverse—as many women can attest from their own ventures in the field. What, apart from childbearing, is the function of the womb? How, then, can giving birth be a dysfunction? The same can be asked of other reproductive functions such as those briefly canvassed in the Introduction: coordinated systems working precisely, if often unsuccessfully, to the end of giving birth.

Pregnancy, childbirth, and allied matters do certainly carry a special emotional charge—sometimes positive, sometimes negative. No emotional reaction should, however, obscure the healthy nature of successful reproductive functioning. A 10-year-old child who is distressed by the onset of puberty should be encouraged to see puberty as a normal human process, not helped to deny or prevent it, or to see dysfunction where none exists. So too with a 15-year-old or 20-year-old or 30-year-old distressed by an unexpected pregnancy—except that here the stakes are very much higher, as another life is involved.

If miscarriage is, as it surely is, reproductive failure, not reproductive success, the same is true of abortion: choice alone cannot turn dysfunction into function, or vice-versa. With no other bodily functions than the reproductive do we so often want to see success or failure, health or disease, as contingent on the mere preferences of individual subjects or 'patients'. Genuine health care must, however, be guided by *health* when responding to requests for interventions; it cannot afford to serve our wishes blindly in invading our bodies whenever we request it[48]—often for reasons which can be separately addressed— and/or the bodies of our children. The right to refuse an intervention and the right to demand one are two very different things: in the one case, but not in the other, our wishes can normally be deferred to without making the doctor a mere tool of harmful, counter-functional requests.[49] All of us do better when our doctors are concerned with us as bodily beings with objective health interests, not just clients with 'choices' uncoupled from our bodies' good functioning.[50]

In striking contrast to the violinist case, continuing (as opposed to terminating) pregnancy support itself constitutes successful physiological functioning for the person who supports. If pregnancy is not a disease, then abortion is not treatment. Pregnancy can certainly be accompanied by medical complications—from minor annoyances to very serious problems which affect the woman's health overall. However, in itself, the presence of a baby in the womb cannot be described as a pathological condition, although it can certainly cause pathological conditions when all is not working as it should.

RIGHT TO CONTROL ONE'S BODY

Of course, many people who accept that pregnancy is a function, not a pathological condition, nonetheless hold that a woman may end her pregnancy at will, since she has a right to avoid parenthood (as discussed above) and/or a right to control her own body. Yet as Christopher Kaczor has noted, if the right to control one's body *means* the right to have an abortion, it cannot be cited as a *reason* why a woman would have a right to an abortion: it is merely a restatement of the claim.[51] Nor is it enough to point to the bodily intimacy of pregnancy and compare this to the intimacy of sex, which must never be imposed.[52] As we shall see in the next chapter, the comparison of rape and non-consensual pregnancy reveals major differences between these, not least because women may and should be protected from unwitting rape (for example, while they are in a coma), though they may not be unwittingly aborted.

If, on the other hand, the right to control one's body means something of more general application, it is simply not the case, as this chapter has attempted to show, that we have unlimited rights over our bodies, particularly when other people's bodies are not only affected but are violently and purposely targeted. There are other situations in life, as we have seen, in which bodily support seems morally mandated. Even more importantly, there is no obvious case in which we are entitled to invade the body of an innocent human being in lethal ways to avoid supporting him or her.

As Mary Catherine Sommers observes, "Precisely because I am embodied, there are few moral obligations I can fulfill without engaging the body."[53] Does recognizing such an obligation in the context of pregnancy involve treating women as incubators or 'fetal containers'? Surely not: if I am a pregnant woman, it is no more treating me as an incubator to expect me to respect my baby's body and allow it to remain within my own than it is treating the baby's father as a cradle to expect him to avoid violent, reckless or negligent treatment of the baby after birth. At least until such time as other carers can take over, it is reasonable to expect those supporting a child to continue to do so, and in any case, to avoid deliberate harm and/or harmful bodily incursions on the child. Just as the parents' own right not to be physically attacked is a 'natural' right that does not require the agreement of others,[54] the same is true of the putative bodily rights of the child they have conceived.

Like men, women have benefited themselves from being gestated when they were babies in the womb. Unlike men, pregnant women are able to benefit their own unborn children in the same way they themselves have been benefited: a way that is needed by every human being, in order for the human race to continue. To withdraw this benefit deliberately from an existing child shows an unwillingness of a rather strong kind to 'give something back'—quite apart from the obvious violence that may be involved in severing the link. Even without admitting a *maternal* link in pregnancy, there are serious presumptive duties to continue such basic support—support towards which one's body is already oriented—and in any case to abstain from violence towards those who are simply living in a place and way reliant on their own and the supporter's normal bodily functions.

In the words of Mary Catherine Sommers, "The parents of the uninvited offspring are morally obligated to sustain him/her only conditionally and temporarily: only what is required for life need be given, only until responsibility can be transferred."[55] But is there more to pregnancy than being a 'good neighbor' or, as Mary Hayden puts it more happily, "the closest neighbor possible . . . the neighbor of the womb"?[56] Pregnancy can clearly lead to (social) parenthood; does it also *constitute* parenthood? And how might that affect the pregnant woman's rights, in addition to her duties? What about serious health problems for her, or other serious problems with her pregnancy? What about the responsibilities of the father, and others? These are issues we will look at in the next chapter, focusing now on pregnancy as 'maternal' support.

NOTES

1 On the relevance of location in U.S. abortion law, see Richard Stith, "Location and Life: How Stenberg v. Carhart Undercut Roe v. Wade", *William and Mary Journal of Women and the Law* 9.2 (2003): 255–78. The focus of this book is not, however, on legal aspects of abortion (or pregnancy more generally). For a historical overview of legal and social aspects of abortion, see John Keown, *Abortion, Doctors and the Law* (Cambridge: Cambridge University Press, 1988); Joseph W. Dellapenna, *Dispelling the Myths of Abortion History* (Durham, North Carolina: Carolina Academic Press, 2006); Ann Farmer, *By Their Fruits: Eugenics, Population Control, and the Abortion Campaign* (Washington: Catholic University of America Press, 2008).

2 The irrelevance of birth to moral status is freely conceded by those authors who regard the unborn baby as also eligible for infanticide after it is born. For a recent presentation of this not-uncommon view in ethics, see note 4 below.

3 This intimacy is sometimes compared to sexual intimacy, and there are some elements in common. However, there are also many differences, not least in relation to the issue of consent (this emerges from consideration of unconscious pregnancy and non-consensual abortion for those unaware of their

pregnancies—an issue explored briefly in the next chapter). Margaret Olivia Little, who makes the comparison ("Abortion, Intimacy, and the Duty to Gestate", *Ethical Theory and Moral Practice* 2 (1999): 295–312), is one of many writers who elide the distinction between a positive duty to aid by gestating (which might be exercised by having one's IVF embryo transferred) and a negative duty not to exercise violence by terminating an existing pregnancy (for another example, see note 7 below).

4   The pain of giving up a baby for adoption has been used to justify, not only social abortion, but social infanticide or 'after-birth abortion', as it has recently been called (Alberto Giubilini, Francesca Minerva, "After-birth Abortion: Why Should the Baby Live?" *Journal of Medical Ethics* 39 (2013): 261–3). Giubilini and Minerva assert that "however weak the interests of actual people can be, they will always trump the alleged interest of potential people to become actual ones, because this latter interest amounts to zero . . . Birthmothers are often reported to experience serious psychological problems due to the inability to elaborate their loss and to cope with their grief. It is true that grief and sense of loss may accompany both abortion and after-birth abortion as well as adoption, but we cannot assume that for the birthmother the latter is the least traumatic".

5   Judith Jarvis Thomson, "A Defense of Abortion", *Philosophy & Public Affairs* 1.1 (1971): 47–66.

6   See, e.g., John Finnis, "The Rights and Wrongs of Abortion: A Reply to Judith Thomson," *Philosophy and Public Affairs* 2.2 (1973): 117–45; Rosalind Hursthouse, *Beginning Lives* (Oxford: Blackwell, 1987), 81–208; Mary Catherine Sommers, "Living Together: Burdensome Pregnancy and the Hospitable Self", in *Abortion: A New Generation of Catholic Responses,* ed. Stephen J. Heaney (Braintree, MA: The Pope John Center, 1992), 243–61; Michael Wreen, "Abortion and Pregnancy Due to Rape", *Philosophia* 21 (1992): 201–20.

The analogy has also attracted much support, including from those who regard both pregnancy and childrearing with a certain repulsion, as the following informal comment illustrates:

"In a college bioethics class, my classmates and I were asked how we would feel if we found ourselves temporarily attached through tubes and wires to another person for almost a year, while he or she depended on us for food and protection. It's a parasitic relationship, we discussed. The host organism gets nothing out of the relationship and is in fact hindered by needing extra nutrients and energy to support the parasite. The lesson was to illustrate how a mother, maybe a rape victim, felt about her unborn and unwanted child.

That hypothetical scenario was the first time I was able to put into words how completely unnatural and abhorrent pregnancy seems to me. To have my body distorted beyond recognition for an alien-looking creature to live there for nine or 10 months and use up my food and energy storage? To have doctors poke and prod at my most private places because that's where it'll be born? Then, to be free of the creature on the inside, but to have to care for it for years and years, while it eats my food, lives in my house, and takes up my energy? A child is a proud role model for any parasite" (Heather Gentry, "No Kids for Me, Thanks: I Don't Enjoy Alien-Parasites", *Slate*, June 12, 2012.

On such 'alienated' approaches to the body, reproductive functioning and parental care, Elena Colombetti makes the following observation:

"Culturally the view has gained ground . . . of human beings as separate individuals in an atomised society. This notion, coupled with a neutral or negative view of the body, has reinforced the techno-scientific model of human action, seen as the instrument and expression of personal choice, or of intentionality envisaged as the sole source of meaning in a neutral or hostile universe" (Elena Colombetti, "Relazione e de-somatizzazione: Per un approccio relazionale al tema della generazione extracorporea", *Medicina e Morale* 62 [2012]: 199).

7 Alex Rajczi rather oddly suggests that the burden of continuing one's pregnancy and giving up the baby for adoption should be compared with the burden of deliberately *becoming* a mother—a commercial surrogate mother—to save the life of a born child who needs expensive surgery (Alex Rajczi, "Abortion, Competing Entitlements, and Parental Responsibility", *Journal of Applied Philosophy* 26 [2009]: 389–90). There are, however, significant differences between meeting the demands of an existing pregnancy, whatever these may be, and assuming a new pregnancy for some purely external, instrumental purpose. On the moral issues raised by surrogacy, see the following two chapters. Rajczi is not alone in blurring the distinction between failure to aid and active withdrawal of aid, often by means that invade another subject and do obvious violence to that subject. It is surprising how often pregnancy is compared to submitting to a new and counter-functional bodily invasion such as organ harvesting.

8 For a frank admission of the violent nature of, in particular, second-trimester abortions, see the comments of one abortion doctor writing in *Reproductive Health Matters*, who describes the harrowing experience of performing an abortion while herself pregnant with a baby of the same gestational age (Lisa H. Harris, "Second Trimester Abortion Provision: Breaking the Silence and Changing the Discourse", *Reproductive Health Matters* 16.31 [2008], Supplement: 74–81). For similar observations by other abortion clinic workers, see www.clinicquotes.com. Violence can, in fact, take different forms: it would be odd to claim that the *method* of bodily attacks or physical incursions on a fetus, if that is the aim of what we do, makes one abortion violent and the other nonviolent. In this respect, at least, it does not matter if a woman takes an abortion pill or a doctor wields an instrument, if what is aimed at is an effect on the body of the fetus of a kind incompatible with life.

This will often be the case, whether or not it is acknowledged that the amniotic sac and placenta are in fact (as they are in origin) fetal tissues. Extraction from the mother will often involve harmful rupture, however achieved, of these and other fetal tissues, even in cases in which it is not also intended that the fetus die (see note 23 below and the discussion of maternal-fetal conflicts in the next chapter).

9 A 'medical' abortion, e.g., using RU486 can have this aim no less than a surgical abortion, despite the fact that in medical abortion the fetus is deliberately attacked 'at one remove' via the woman taking the drug. Whether using a morning-after pill pre-implantation necessarily involves an intention to kill the embryo (if one should be conceived) or to otherwise affect its body or rather 'simply' involves the intention to refuse to nurture it by making the uterus a hostile environment is a question I will not pursue here. The morning-after pill also, of course, raises questions explored in this chapter concerning pregnancy as 'basic support'.

10 Finnis, "The Rights and Wrongs of Abortion", 140.

11 Nicholas Denyer, "Is Anything Absolutely Wrong?" in *Human Lives: Critical Essays on Consequentialist Bioethics*, eds. David S. Oderberg and Jacqueline A. Laing (London: Palgrave Macmillan, 1997), 39–57.

12 Christopher Kaczor, "Notes and Abstracts," *National Catholic Bioethics Quarterly* 11 (2011): 581. Kaczor is perhaps conceding too much in saying that continuation of pregnancy (as opposed, perhaps, to some cases of

commencement of pregnancy) involves, like donating a kidney, a 'partial violation of bodily integrity' (580–1). He is, however, right to say that "A fortiori, if people have a right to bodily integrity and so do not have a duty to donate a kidney, then people in utero have a right not to have their bodily integrity fatally violated by abortion. No one should be forced to donate a kidney to save a human life, so it is even more obvious that no fetal person should have his or her bodily integrity violated in a lethal manner so that someone else can avoid continuing to be a gestational mother" (580).

13 The connection between pregnancy and parenthood, and pregnancy and sexual acts, will be explored in more detail in the next two chapters. In this chapter, the focus is more on rights and duties of a kind which could apply to all pregnancies, including those resulting from coercion and/or non-sexual acts such as transfer of IVF embryos.

14 Thomson, "A Defense of Abortion", 59. A very different approach to an unexpected pregnancy, though one expressed using similar imagery, can be seen in the words of Isabelle de Mezerac, the mother of a child later found to have a lethal anomaly:
     "The idea that I could possibly be pregnant seemed impossible. I was dragging my feet at this renewed prospect: to start it all over, diapers, baby bottles, sleepless nights. But it also meant reliving first smiles, first words, and first steps and savoring the complete abandonment newborns have in the arms of their parents. Little by little, the perspective that was drawn on the horizon began to take form in my head; my heart was already endeared by this little one who had forced through our door." Isabelle de Mezerac, *Un enfant pour l'eternite* (Paris: Editions du Rocher, 2004), cit. Amy Kuebelbeck and Deborah L. Davis, *A Gift of Time: Continuing Your Pregnancy when your Baby's Life Is Expected to Be Brief* (Baltimore: The Johns Hopkins University Press, 2011), 2–3.

15 While Thomson comments disapprovingly on those who see the pregnant woman as a mere 'house' (52–3), she herself uses property analogies in a way that disturbs at least one feminist critic:
     "An analysis of Thomson's examples and analogies reveals a consistent theory of property rights and the body as property. This theory holds that the terms of possession, the use, development and disposal of property are unconditionally under the control of the possessor. The body is compared to the house (the archetypal American property, defensible in the myths by the gun-toting patriarch): the house sealed contraceptively against fetal invasion; the house invaded and blown up along with its maternal inhabitant by the fetal invader; the house which, when all is said and done, is owned by the mother." Sommers, "Living Together", 245.
     If the body is me, I do not own my body in the way I own my house: as I claim in the next chapter, human beings are not property, not even of themselves.

16 For a discussion of this point, see Steven L. Ross, "Abortion and the Death of the Fetus," *Philosophy & Public Affairs* 11 (1982): 232–24.

17 See E. S. Draper, Z. Alfirevic et al., "An investigation into the reporting and management of late terminations of pregnancy (between 22 +0 and 26 +6 weeks of gestation) within NHS Hospitals in England in 2006: the EPICure preterm cohort study," *BJOG: An International Journal of Obstetrics and Gynaecology* 119 (2012), published online 7 March 2012, at DOI: 10.1111/j.1471–0528.2012.03285.x. The study authors note that "Dealing with a liveborn infant following a TOP [termination of pregnancy] is extremely stressful for all involved. The UK RCOG [Royal College of Obstetricians and Gynaecologists] guidance recommends that feticide is routinely offered for TOPs for fetal

abnormality after 21+6 weeks of gestation . . . High rates of feticide were achieved in accordance with the guidance. In a small number of places parents were noted to have refused feticide; however, it is not clear why in the remaining cases feticide had not been carried out, or whether it had been offered" (4).

18 Bertha Alvarez Manninen helpfully notes that there are "three ways to interpret the nature of the abortion right. First, the right can be interpreted as a mechanism to prevent unwanted social parenthood. Second, [it] can be interpreted as a mechanism to prevent unwanted genetic parenthood . . . Third, the right to an abortion can be interpreted as an instance of the broader right to bodily autonomy qua the right not to be subjected to unwanted bodily intrusion" (Bertha Alvarez Manninen, "Rethinking Roe V. Wade: Defending the Abortion Right in the Face of Contemporary Opposition," *American Journal of Bioethics* 10.12 [2010]: 36). Manninen then observes of genetic parenthood—though failing to apply this to the offspring immediately after conception—"While exercising this right entails that you can *prevent the existence* of a genetically related child, it does not entail that you can *kill* an already existing genetically related child if you decide, **after her birth** [emphasis added] that you no longer wish to be a parent" (37).

19 Infanticide is defended by some ethicists today (see note 4 of this chapter) and was not uncommon in the ancient world. In Rome, for example, newborn babies (often in practice female or disabled babies) could be killed at the behest of not their mother but their father.

20 It may be objected that the man's part in conceiving a child and (perhaps) supporting the woman through her pregnancy is very much less than the woman's in terms of time and effort invested. While this is normally true, it is not clear why it should be relevant to deliberate life termination. Do parents who have conceived a child with great difficulty (say, after costly attempts to reverse male or female sterilisation) have greater powers of life and death over the child than those who have not faced these difficulties? Do these powers of life and death last into the child's toddlerhood? If not, why not?

No amount of effort invested in conceiving or nurturing a child can turn that child into property, though it may compound the parents' sense of loss— and perhaps their actual loss in a certain sense—if the child should die. Such 'investment' may be one way in which one particular homicide may be worse than another (as discussed in the previous chapter)—though in a different way, it can be worse that a child has not even lived long enough to attract such an investment. Interestingly, if we are to count investment not only of parents, but of remote ancestors, many of whom will have hoped for descendants, there is an odd corollary: since homicide in the 21st century destroys the investment of so many more ancestors, it might be worse than homicide in the 12th (Coope, *Worth and Welfare*, 141). Yet if this is so, it is surely not because people in the 12th century had a lower moral *status* than our own; rather, such investment-frustration would be simply one more way in which the basic wrong of homicide could be exacerbated.

21 See also Lee, *Abortion and Unborn Human Life*, 136: "Being dead is not the same as never having been; otherwise not procreating, would be equivalent to killing. Being deprived of life by someone from whom I received life is still being deprived of life and thus being seriously harmed". In similar vein, Kaczor talks about wanting the baby dead, observing moderately:

"Surely this desire to kill one's offspring ought not to be gratified. There are men with similar desires, desires that could only be satisfied by killing the child. In some cases, such a man will have created a new human being with a woman who does not share his desires and so refuses to get an abortion. For men, the right to gratify the desire not to continue to be a genetic parent does not justify abortion, since this would interfere with the bodily integrity of the mother, but it rather justifies infanticide. Indeed, the 'right not to be a genetic parent' exercised after one has already become a genetic parent, leads to a denial of the right to life of even adult children" (Kaczor, Notes and Abstracts, 584–5).

22 Manninen, "Rethinking Roe V. Wade", 38.

23 To be more specific, I am intending to cut through 'this', where 'this' is known to be the living body of an innocent human being. In a similar way, an abortion doctor may be intending not just to remove 'this' but to remove 'this' in pieces (bearing in mind that 'this' will include parts of the fetus such as the amniotic sac and placenta). The doctor cannot, at any rate, intend to remove the fetus whole while knowing all along that the abortion method used involves removing it in pieces.

On the relationship between the intention to invade or otherwise manipulate the fetus and the (separable, contingent) intention to end life, see the discussion in the next chapter. Note that in the case of induced labor pre-viability, if the fetus has not been lethally injected beforehand it may well be killed by the contractions themselves. Where the woman's body itself is used in this way by the doctor as a means to extract the fetus, exerting immediate pressure of a kind intended and/or known to threaten its life, it is difficult to argue that this is less violent than manually pulling out the fetus, where such targeted pulling is similarly not unlikely itself to cause death.

24 Cf. Coope: "It is natural to talk of sanctity of life when we are thinking of the teaching that we are not to lay our murderous hands upon one another. By contrast, the idea of value seems more apposite when talking about the duty to rescue. This is because the notion of costs is here relevant. We are not to count the costs of respecting the sanctity of life, at least where this is narrowly construed: that is part of what we have in mind by talking about sanctity in such matters. But it is perfectly reasonable to consider the cost even in a purely monetary sense, when thinking whom to save. This is a regular part of public health care. And we will reasonably be prepared to spend more saving some rather than others, thus regarding some as 'more worth saving' for one reason or another. Someone might be inclined to express this by talking about their differing value, though we might not find such language comfortable, or even particularly intelligible. However when we think of the sanctity of their lives, we will think them all alike. They will have an inviolability which does not differ in degree" (Coope, *Worth and Welfare*, 61–2).

25 Choosing harm by passive means applies more to the case of the infant who could be left unfed and untended with the aim of bringing about its death than to the fetus who does not normally need 'positive acts' (or at least, *chosen* positive acts) on the woman's part over and above her everyday activities in order to survive. It is, however, possible to imagine a case where the woman declines (say) anti-miscarriage treatment, not out of fears or concerns related to the treatment itself, but precisely in order to enable the miscarriage.

26 Mullin observes: "Unwanted pregnancy, even without its added moral dimension, is . . . far more of a violation of a person's autonomy and sense of self than forced labor, and, like childrearing, there are no respites from its demands and its transformations of a woman's life . . . There are many experiences, some of them also involving radical change—such as arduous and risky travel, mountaineering, and becoming involved as a social activist in places experiencing war, poverty, or civil strife—that people take on voluntarily. This is, of course, no argument for forcing people who have not sought out these experiences to climb mountains, parachute from airplanes, trek across deserts, or toil in dangerous situations" (70).

Leaving aside the vexed issue of military conscription, we should note that all these examples are of (a) private projects of no significant value to others or (b) projects for the benefit of strangers, not one's own kin. Care for a newborn child or disabled family member—which can also be an overwhelming, highly stressful and life-changing experience—would be a closer comparison. We might think, for example, of parents of an autistic child who are desperate for a respite: no one would argue that such parents may seek relief by killing their child, though all of us would (or should) sympathise and help them if we can.

27 Lee, *Abortion and Unborn Human Life*, 126–8.

28 Imagine a woman who is very tempted to have an abortion due to unusually burdensome circumstances, but is fortified by considering her own mother's very difficult pregnancy. Of course, those who have not been willingly nurtured by others can still have nurturing duties themselves: an abandoned toddler is not thereby justified in abandoning her own toddler when she grows up.

29 On the question of moral absolutism, see Nicholas Denyer, "Is Anything Absolutely Wrong?"

30 This point would presumably be accepted by Thomson: "I am not claiming that people have a right to do anything whatever to save their lives. I think, rather, that there are drastic limits to the right of self-defense. If someone threatens you with death unless you torture someone to death, I think you have not the right, even to save your life, to do so." ("A Defense of Abortion", 53.) Thomson goes on, however, to draw a sharp distinction between such cases and those where there are only two people involved, the innocent threat and the threatened person, where she believes the latter may defend him/herself against the former.

31 We can imagine that the Secret Police demand to be presented with the corpse as the price of letting the parent go free.

32 Both she and the father have duties to themselves in this regard, not only to the child: abortion may have seriously harmful effects on them, quite apart from its effects on the baby. Unlike the risks of pregnancy, which perhaps sometimes cannot be avoided morally once a pregnancy has begun (though see the next chapter on high-risk situations), the risks of abortion are entirely avoidable unless there is a *duty* to abort in some situations, which most abortion advocates would not claim (see, however, Lara Denis, "A Kantian Approach to Abortion", *Philosophy and Phenomenological Research* 76.1 (2008): 132). On the psychological impact of abortion, see P. K. Coleman, "Abortion and Mental Health: Quantitative Synthesis and Analysis of Research Published 1995–2009", *British Journal of Psychiatry* 199 (2011): 180–6; D. M. Ferguson, L. J. Horwood, and J. M. Boden, "Abortion and Mental Health Disorders: Evidence from a 30 Year Longitudinal Study", *British Journal of Psychiatry* 193 (2008): 444–51; David M. Ferguson, L. John Horwood, and Joseph M. Boden, "Does Abortion Reduce the Mental Health Risks of Unwanted or Unintended Pregnancy? A Reappraisal of the Evidence", *Australian and New Zealand Journal of Psychiatry*, found at: DOI: 10.1177/0004867413484597, published online 3 April 2013; Carlo V. Bellieni and Giuseppe Buonocore, "Abortion and Subsequent Mental Health: Review of the Literature", *Psychiatry and Clinical Neurosciences* 67.5 (2013): 301–10. For more anecdotal accounts, see e.g. Melinda Tankard Reist, Giving Sorrow Words: Women's Stories of Grief After Abortion (Sydney: Duffy & Snellgrove, 2000). Self-harm is, at least on some views of ethics, no less a moral concern than harm to other people, even if refraining from self-protective actions cannot always be fairly so categorized. And while wrongful moral choices can generally be seen as 'self-harming', there is arguably a particular harm and deprivation involved in harm to one's offspring, in whose welfare one has a role-related stake.

33 Patrick Lee observes that "His [the father's] duty does not involve as direct a bodily relationship with the child as the mother's, but it may be equally or even more burdensome. In certain circumstances, his obligation to care for the child (and the child's mother) and especially his obligation to provide financial support, may severely limit his freedom and even require months or, indeed, years, of extremely burdensome physical labour." (Lee, *Abortion and Unborn Human Life*, 129–30). In regard to legal duties of child support, David Boonin is, however, right to point out that the State does not directly constrain the man to work at a particular task, but simply requires him to support his child in some way when they live apart (Boonin, *A Defense of Abortion*, 251) (though perhaps, we might add, in more specific ways such as bottle feeding when the child is in the man's care). Such duties must, in any case, be distinguished from the negative duty not to cause the child harm, such as via physical assaults. On the postnatal duties of parents towards their children, see the next two chapters.

34 Anna Smajdor, "The Moral Imperative for Ectogenesis", *Cambridge Quarterly of Healthcare Ethics* 16 (2007): 337: "In short, what is required is ectogenesis: the development of artificial wombs that can sustain foetuses to term without the need for women's bodies. Only by thus remedying the natural or physical injustices involved in the unequal gender roles of reproduction can we alleviate the social injustices that arise from them." See also Smajdor's follow-up paper "In Defence of Ectogenesis," *Cambridge Quarterly of Healthcare Ethics* 21 (2012): 90–103.

35 Sommers, "Living Together", 250.

36 Of course, negative duties not to harm are similarly linked to capabilities—here for harming and for making harmful choices. It makes no sense to talk of the duties of babies, who can neither choose to harm, nor choose not to harm.

37 Cf. Christopher Coope: "If justice, in the sense of what is owed, lays a burden on someone, it is not always a burden which it is entirely that individual's own affair to carry . . . some of the 'owings' under justice are simply visited upon us, and may be severe. A child, let us say, suddenly demands care quite beyond what is usual on account of its unexpectedly acquired disabilities. Justice suddenly demands that one changes one's whole life. One has to take on a different role, become a different person, lay aside cherished prospects. Could it not also be a requirement of justice that others rally round—either as individuals directly or through public institutions?" (Coope, *Worth and Welfare*, 5).

38 In pregnancy, the mother's organs do support the baby, as well as her own body; however, it would be rash indeed to claim that this is no part of their function. Such a claim would leave the reproductive organs isolated as the *only* maternal organs geared to supporting a child—despite the fact that they would be quite unable to achieve this without the help of other parts of the woman's body. In contrast, with conjoined twins, not a single organ of either twin is *functionally* oriented towards the conjoined state, however much that state may have 'co-opted' normal healthy human functions. The same would, of course, be true of male pregnancy should this ever be achieved: a (necessarily) ectopic pregnancy in a man would have even less claim than ectopic pregnancy in a woman to involve functional support—or at least some elements of such support.

39 "Abortion, if it is an act of control, is a violent act of control. When a woman is pregnant, be it six days or six months, her body has become inextricably wedded to the body of another living being; the only way out of that relationship for a woman who does not want to be pregnant is a violent one, an act that destroys the fetus and invades the body—and often the mind— of his or her mother." Anne M. Maloney, "Cassandra's Fate: Why Feminists Ought to Be Pro-Life", in *Abortion: A New Generation of Catholic Responses*, ed.

Stephen J. Heaney (Braintree, MA: The Pope John Center, 1992), 213. Cf. Wolf-Devine and Devine: "All too often, people avoid looking at the concrete reality of abortion—either the details of the procedure or the physical characteristics of the unborn. The desire to distance oneself from the physical reality is intensely felt here in a way it is not in the case of other medical procedures. From the point of view of a woman, the abortion procedure is invasive in a peculiarly intimate way, as even many pro-choice women have noted." Wolf-Devine and Devine, "A Communitarian Pro-Life Perspective," 76.

40 Adult humans have a function of carrying, if not a function of being carried. In contrast, with breastfeeding and pregnancy the functioning goes very much both ways.

41 Again, we need to distinguish between any positive obligations we may have to choose to support (e.g., deliberately to *assume* support, or to take positive measures to *continue* support) and in contrast, any *negative* obligations to refrain from harmful targeting of those whom we believe, whether rightly or wrongly, we are not obliged to support.

42 As I argue in the next two chapters, this is so even if the fetus is not the woman's genetic child, as with gestational surrogacy and/or egg donation. Once maternal functioning has been engaged, the fetus belongs functionally and relationally with its (gestational) mother.

43 As Beckwith points out, "Burglars don't belong in other people's homes, whereas preborn children belong in *no other place except* their mother's womb" (Beckwith, *Defending Life*, 273). With ectopic pregnancy, the child will, however, have implanted elsewhere in the woman's body. Here terms like "blundering" can indeed be applied to either party to this terrible 'shared blunder': the embryo is functioning temporarily, but in a highly abnormal place that threatens the functioning of the woman even as it partially co-opts it. On this and other medical maternal-fetal conflicts, see the next chapter.

44 David Boonin appears to conflate these in his comments on the fetus being in the 'right place' (*A Defense of Abortion*, 245).

45 Maloney, "Cassandra's Fate", 212–13. Elsewhere ("You Say You Want a Revolution?" 38–39) Maloney says that:
"The ethic of abortion on demand espoused by both Androgynous Idealists and Woman Idealists actually tells women that they simply cannot be the equals of men unless they chemically or surgically alter their bodies to *be* more like male bodies. The clear implication is that there is something *wrong* with the female body as it is naturally, that it needs fixing somehow. The ethic of abortion encourages (nay, insists) that women must sever their traditional tendency to invest themselves sexually only in relationships that promise commitment and longevity, to take care to offer themselves only to those they can trust with their deepest vulnerabilities. When contraception fails (as all forms do), the abortion ethic offers the woman the "choice" to have her body surgically invaded and her unborn child torn from her womb so that she will not have to lose a day in the public, competitive world—the male world. Yet the holders of the abortion ethic call themselves feminist, and attempt to silence their sisters who disagree." See also Wolf-Devine and Devine, "A Communitarian Pro-Life Perspective", 108–9.

46 Mary Rosera Joyce, "Are Women Controlling Their Own Minds? The Power of Puritan and Playboy Mentalities", in *Abortion: A New Generation of Catholic Responses*, ed. Stephen J. Heaney (Braintree, MA: The Pope John Center, 1992), 232.

47 Smajdor, "The Moral Imperative for Ectogenesis", 343.

48 Admittedly, there are cosmetic, nonmedical interventions which may still be morally permissible for doctors to perform—though only on the assumption that no harm (or no serious permanent harm) is done to those involved. On

health care and respect for health, see Watt, "Life and Health: A Value in Itself for Human Beings?"

49   Note that the request is for a bodily invasion, and is thus particularly hard to justify, if we accept the intuition that we are particularly responsible for harm we cause by deliberate bodily movements—above all where the body-space of others is deliberately invaded. *Abstention* from bodily invasion, in contrast, can be justified where the invasion will be harmful or where, although potentially beneficial, it is unwanted by the patient, as with unwanted cesarean sections (bearing in mind that the doctor is failing to treat many other women in the world besides those refusing treatment). Of course, if a doctor were *intending harm* by withholding (say) cesarian sections from patients who needed them, this too would be unconscionable: people can be wrongfully targeted by omission, as well as by 'positive acts'.

50   This would also apply to counter-functional attempts to *initiate* a pregnancy, such as futuristic attempts to initiate ectopic pregnancy in a man (or in a woman without a womb who wishes to become pregnant).

51   Kaczor, Notes and Abstracts, 583.

52   See note 3 of this chapter.

53   Sommers, "Living Together", 247.

54   See Hursthouse, *Beginning Lives,* 199.

55   Sommers, "Living Together", 255.

56   "Humanness is the same whether found in a fetus or in an adult. Thus, since abortion involves the refusal to love another's humanness, it also involves the refusal to love oneself . . . one cannot hate her indwelling offspring and still properly love herself and her neighbors. Does not abortion involve killing the closest neighbor possible, i.e., the neighbor of the womb? Moreover, abortion kills the closest possible likeness of self, that is one's own child" (Mary Hayden, "The 'Feminism' of Aquinas' Natural Law: Relationships, Love and New Life", in *Abortion: A New Generation of Catholic Responses,* ed. Stephen J. Heaney [Braintree, Mass: The Pope John Center, 1992], 241).

3 The Maternal Pregnancy

Does being or becoming pregnant make one a *mother*, we can ask at this point in our reflections, or just a helpful assisting adult? —at least in cases where motherhood is not deliberately assumed. This question has important practical implications, which are perhaps best approached by beginning with *rights conferred* by pregnancy on the woman: rights that are difficult to understand if pregnancy is, or can be, simply a generous—a particularly generous—way of being neighborly towards a child in need. The neighbor, or mere neighbor, approach seems inadequate when these *rights to mother* are seriously considered: the child either is, or risks being, or is perhaps appropriately,[1] more to the woman socially and emotionally than that.

BECOMING PREGNANT: RIGHTS CONFERRED

In looking at the duties involved in pregnancy and childbirth, the rights these confer are often forgotten. These rights do not seem limited to the right to act as a temporary 'good neighbor', important as that is. As we shall see, this applies to the question of surrogacy and the forced relinquishment of the baby to the commissioning couple: such a move seems to violate genuine maternal rights on the part of surrogate *mothers*, as they are often called. The 'right to mother' also applies to the question of forced destruction of a child in utero: if an abortion is literally forced on a woman, this is not only a violent invasion which kills a human being inside her (though that sounds horrible enough) but an invasion which kills what is in fact her own offspring—here quite against her will. To take seriously the moral wrong involved, we need to take seriously the woman's *maternal* relationship with what is destroyed, and that applies even in cases where the woman is unaware of what is going on.

PREGNANCY AND ABORTION IN COMATOSE WOMEN

To carry out an abortion on an unconscious woman who does not know that she is pregnant[2] seems to violate existing maternity, and to be an egregious assault on the woman for that reason. A woman in a coma who is pregnant, whether after earlier consensual intercourse, or after the particular outrage of rape,[3] seems to have acquired maternal rights, though rights of which she is unaware. To claim instead that 'unconscious pregnancy' is itself a morally intolerable bodily invasion raises the question whether non-consensual abortion of a comatose woman should be mandatory, just as we would prevent such a woman from being raped. True, the imposition of pregnancy by rape,[4] and thus its later presence, is very much part of the moral offence of the rapist. The right not to be made pregnant while one is unconscious[5] cannot even be waived, any more than the right not to be raped while one is unconscious: there are rights over our own bodies that we simply cannot waive.[6] (It may seem unnecessary to state this; however, at least one writer has seriously proposed that women might sign advance directives allowing themselves to be used as surrogate mothers should they fall into a 'persistent vegetative state.')[7]

Notwithstanding the fact that the right not to be made pregnant while one is unconscious is inalienable, it is, it can be argued, the abortion of such pregnancies,[8] not their sheer continuation, which violates the woman's bodily integrity, as well as her baby's, in a truly intolerable way.[9] Not every effect of a violation itself violates: think of the baby's passage through the birth canal to be born or indeed, its attempting to breastfeed if placed on the mother's breast. The violent act that caused the presence of the child is in the past and cannot now be undone; the presence of the child can indeed be 'erased', but not without harm and injustice to both parties. An abortion would in fact be a new invasive act, fully avoidable, which would make the woman's own invaded body the unwitting site of a violent invasion of her child's.

Abortion seems, on this description, no more defensible where the woman is unconscious than where she is actively resisting the abortion—or indeed, where she is consenting, though often with reluctance, to have the life within her destroyed. In the case of abortion following rape, the violent destruction of the rapist's (innocent) child is also the destruction of the woman's own child (we will return shortly to the issue of rape pregnancy, where the woman's relationship with the rape-conceived baby is often presumed to be non-maternal: a presumption at odds, as we will see, with the experience of many women who find themselves in that situation).

THE RIGHT TO MOTHER

Quite generally, and without in any way excluding rape pregnancies, which carry the same rights, it is very important to recognize the raft of rights that pregnancy confers on the pregnant woman, over and above her right to continue her pregnancy[10]—from the right of the competent woman to be the 'guardian' of the pregnancy in regard to (for example) food, drink and consent to medical treatments for herself and the fetus to her right to keep and raise the child when it is born.[11] If a pregnant woman is just a 'good neighbor' to the fetus, it is difficult to see why she would have such a strong presumptive right to keep and raise the child. After all, foster-carers of new-born babies do not necessarily acquire the right to parent them indefinitely just by caring for them—and of course, bonding with them—for weeks or even months after birth. While it is arguable that the rights of foster-carers to keep babies should be better acknowledged after some time has passed, it is interesting to see how ready many of us are to acknowledge the birth mother's right to claim back her child, even after many weeks' separation, and despite the fact that her postnatal 'social parenthood' may be practically non-existent. This is not just a question of genetics, as we may attribute such rights also to genetically unrelated 'surrogate' mothers (so-called 'gestational carriers')—even in the teeth of competing claims of both genetic parents.

Why do we feel such qualms about seizing a baby from a birth mother who wants to keep her child, even if she was not intending motherhood (or not envisaged as such) in conceiving or gestating? What is it about pregnancy and childbirth that gives a woman *rights to mother*—even if, so many of us believe, the child has a prior mother in the form of the woman providing the ovum? (We will come later to the question of fathers, but let us stay on that of mothers for the moment.)

It may be objected that the surrogate mother, unlike the woman who is pregnant unexpectedly, did at least *choose* to be pregnant, so has acquired maternal rights by choice, at least to that extent. However, she, unlike the commissioning couple, did not choose to enter into a parental relationship acknowledged as such; on the contrary, she specifically undertook to sign over to the couple her parental rights (or the parental rights she would otherwise have had, at least in legal terms). Nonetheless, to commandeer the baby at birth against the wishes of the surrogate mother seems a serious moral wrong, and something quite different from taking the baby from a wet-nurse or foster-mother who wants to keep the child. This suggests that the surrogate 'mother' is indeed a mother, if she has such an overriding right to keep any child born. It seems that something about pregnancy—if only (implausibly) the end-stage of pregnancy when the baby passes through and *leaves* her body—has made the surrogate a mother with genuine maternal rights. Moreover, any earlier attempt to waive these maternal rights by signing a surrogacy contract, refusing to call herself a mother and so on are clearly unavailing, if she may choose to keep the baby at this later stage. Admittedly, she may choose instead to relinquish the child—though this may nor may not be the best choice morally, depending on her circumstances, the recipient couple's suitability, their genetic link, if any, with the child and so on. However, the right that the surrogate is waiving is a genuine maternal right; moreover, this right cannot be waived while she is still pregnant with the baby, and hence inevitably acting as a mother[12]—a gestational mother— to it. She may choose after birth to waive her 'right to mother', in favor of the commissioning couple or another couple; however, she may not choose to waive this right before birth in a way that will bind her after birth. Moreover, there is a sense (as we shall see) in which a birth mother is *always* the (or a) mother of the child, with latent maternal rights and duties that may be reactivated at a later time.

ALL ROLES CHOSEN?

Is the maternal role, alternatively, something always chosen or contractual, as is sometimes suggested? This seems implausible: to begin with, it is clearly *not* the case that the role can *simply* be chosen by those who want to parent some particular child. After all, it is the surrogate herself, not her flatmate, however emotionally involved she may be, whose wish to parent the baby we respect and respond to. If maternity were purely a matter of states of mind, it would be enough for the flatmate to declare herself the mother—perhaps in especially forcible terms—and demand to keep the child when it is born. Even if the flatmate engineered the whole situation (say, by persuading her friend to take on surrogacy work), to talk about "mental conception"[13] as opposed to would-be motherhood in her case seems perverse. If 'choice' is thought to be necessary for motherhood, it is certainly not thought to be sufficient.

More generally, we do not tend to see most family roles[14] as a matter of contingent choice. On the contrary, one of the *advantages* many of us see in family roles[15] is precisely their 'givenness': unlike many other kinds of role, they are precisely *not* contingent on prior agreement, at least in many cases. Admittedly, both marriage and adoption *are* initially voluntary, though 'locking' one into the new relationship from that point: family roles can therefore be chosen in some cases, if not readily unchosen. And, of course, many choose to 'try for a baby,' or at least, to allow the possibility of conception— although many others do not. Having said that, the roles of child, grandchild or sibling,[16] which can also carry important rights and duties, are clearly not chosen by the children, grandchildren or (younger)[17] siblings concerned. There is a value—a particular appropriateness—attached to promoting a family member's welfare, even if some unrelated person could in theory offer similar support.

Prenatal bonding does not always occur, but many of us think of it as somehow appropriate; thus we are disturbed when surrogate mothers report making an effort, whether successful or otherwise, to avoid bonding with the baby. Others claim that they do not have to try,[18] and may describe themselves as 'carriers', 'incubators' or 'hotels' for housing babies[19] —the babies of others, as they see it.[20] Yet surely, here the surrogate is in effect (to return to the themes of Chapter 1) treating her pregnant body and thus her very self as a subpersonal instrument—or at least, seriously devaluing what she/her body does in pregnancy. She is not treating her ability to gestate a child as bearing a unique and even sublime interpersonal meaning. Just as prostitution is a radical impoverishment of sex, surrogacy seems a radical impoverishment of pregnancy, in treating the bodily 'housing' of a child in such an impersonal and pragmatic way.[21] Even those surrogates who are anxiously devoted to the welfare of 'the couple's' baby are failing in their very devotion to appreciate their own rights and duties as what are accurately called gestational *mothers* —not just 'carriers' or carers.[22] And as for the claim sometimes made that a surrogate has a right to keep the baby if she wishes, but simply as a 'product' of her 'gestational labor',[23] the question arises how nurturing a child, in or outside the womb, can make it one's property (that, after all, is the connotation here)[24] as opposed to one's responsibility.

Of course, acknowledging the parental significance of gestation is in no way to deny that genetic and social relationships are *also* genuinely parental. If surrogates are parents, so too are donors of sperm and ova (certainly, in the view of some at least of their offspring)[25] and above all, those who 'parent' children for years and even decades after birth. Social parenthood is in many ways the most important aspect of parenthood, and the point to which all other forms are ideally tending. However, even those who lay most stress on the social aspect of parenthood will normally concede that gestation and genetics have *some* significance: babies should not (for example) be randomly allocated to women who have just given birth.[26] Admittedly, if babies have already been separated from their birth mothers for many months, the most recent provider of 'caring input' will sometimes have a better claim than the earlier provider, if continuity of commitment and fidelity to roles has value for bonding and for the child's sense of identity. It is not good for children to be passed from mother to mother when this can be avoided. Yet for that very reason, it seems difficult to deny that the woman who has just had a baby is precisely—even archetypically—mother to that child. It is she who has been acting as the baby's mother for the past nine months—and, in most cases, bonding psychologically and not 'only' biologically. There are, of course, exceptions: the comatose woman, for example, who wakes to find herself a mother will have no experience of bonding, or of the various strains of pregnancy that may either hinder or promote this.[27] Nonetheless, she *is*, I am claiming, mother to the child she gives birth to, of whom she may not be deprived—not even by the child's genetic mother— unless she is truly unable or unwilling to care for the child herself.

Nor is this just a matter of general causal responsibility: the duties of existing surrogate and/or genetic mothers differ significantly from those of IVF scientists who create embryos, despite the latter's heavy causal involvement in those embryos' production. Such scientists may well have responsibilities to the embryos once created, such as to encourage the genetic mother to gestate her 'spare' embryos left in the freezer. However, a female IVF scientist would not have a duty to gestate the embryos herself, however copiously and even recklessly she may have brought them into being. Nor, indeed, would she have a *right* to gestate the embryos: whatever her other responsibilities for them, these are simply not her embryos. In contrast, women and men who conceive non-voluntarily can be thought of as having real parental responsibilities, and this applies as much to male victims of 'sperm-napping'[28] as it does to female victims of rape or other non-consensual impregnation.

Pregnancy is not just *a* way but *the* archetypal, timeless way in which a child is socially 'placed', both in terms of its origin and in terms of its destiny and expectations for its care. The expectation that birth mothers keep their children, defeasible as this expectation may be, gives a certain security to the woman, the child, other family and those about them. Origin matters for the child's sense of identity: it not only answers some questions for the child about his or her psychophysical makeup[29]—or helps to lay these questions to rest—but carries an important message about parental acceptance and the 'givenness' of family roles. As we shall see, all being well, pregnancy has a complex social meaning not just for immediate family but for wider society, which is impoverished when aspects of maternity—or indeed, paternity—are separated out and allocated to different people. (The role of pregnancy in linking a child publicly not just with a particular woman, but also with a particular man in certain circumstances will be explored in the next chapter.)

ACKNOWLEDGING MATERNITY: PREGNANCY AND BIRTH AFTER RAPE

What role, then, remains for the woman's own acceptance of her maternity? Surrogate mothers routinely refuse to accept that they are mothers—which is of course the very nature of their contract. Some contracts explicitly require that the surrogate mother not attempt to form a maternal relationship with the child,[30] and all require or expect her to relinquish the child when it is born. More generally, some women who are not surrogate mothers refuse to acknowledge (or fully acknowledge) not only their maternity but the very existence of their pregnancy—particularly if there is some accompanying trauma. Even childbirth can be emotionally denied, even when it is intellectually accepted. Wholly understandable as this reaction may be in certain very painful situations, to deny the reality of childbirth and motherhood will not, of course, make them go away. Here is one first-hand account provided many years later by a victim of rape which resulted in conception. "Connie Sellars" is describing herself as a 15-year-old girl giving birth to the baby so conceived:

> [T]he denial was so strong that I asked to be blindfolded in the delivery room so I wouldn't have any visual memories of the birth. (Now

any woman who has given birth knows that there must be pretty strong denial if you can go through labor and still deny there is a baby involved.)

I was able to deny my motherhood until I heard my baby's cry. Then I knew I was a mother. I kept on the blindfold but I wanted to know if he was healthy and what sex he was. I had a son.

I truly believe that God has given women hormones that cause them to love their babies. Love them enough that they will get up in the middle of the night and care for the baby's needs at the expense of their own. By the next morning, I wanted to see my baby, but I tried to resist. After two days I asked to see him, feed him, hold him, and say goodbye.

They let us go into a room all to ourselves with a rocking chair. I had never held such a small baby but it came naturally. I fed him and held him for a very long time. I told him I loved him but couldn't keep him. I told him that his birth was not his fault. I told him to be a good little boy and make some family very happy.[31]

One of the many striking things about this story is what seems the appropriateness of this very young girl acknowledging her maternity at the very point when she is relinquishing her child to other parents. Bonding is not, in her account, the *source*, but the *result*, of her motherhood, with which she now fully identifies, though her plans for her baby are unchanged.[32] The decision to relinquish the child to other parents is hers to make, for the very reason that pregnancy—at the very least, the culmination of pregnancy in childbirth—has made her the mother of a child for whom she is morally (and legally) responsible. It is not her emotional response that makes "Connie Sellers" a mother; rather, she identifies herself as having been 'in denial' before this point of a motherhood that was none the less real before it was acknowledged. And while Connie refers to herself before the birth as being "soon to be a mother",[33] it is clear that, at any rate, she now believes the fetus she was carrying was the same individual as her born child: "If I had taken his life", she says, "there would have been no good".[34]

For Connie, the emotional change happened after birth, while for some raped women the emotional acknowledgement of their maternal link with the baby—a link they see, again, as predating that acknowledgement—came many months before. Thus Mary Murray comments:

In the early months of the pregnancy, I was anxious. I did not know how to feel about the baby; it was different than with my other girls. But as I began to feel life, I fell in love with my baby. I had forgotten that she was *my* child too. Once I realized that, I began to feel excited about the birth, although I did worry about "bad genes", how the baby would look (the rapist was black, I was white), what people would say, etc.[35]

In contrast, Sharon "Bailey" testifies of her rape-conceived child, whom she nonetheless counts as one of her own children:

> As for feelings about her while I was pregnant, I don't recall having any. I thought when she kicked, etc., that it was exciting, but I didn't have deep mother instincts. Basically my feelings were, "it's just you and me, kid". I considered us both to be victims. Kind of like the bond between hostages.[36]

Later, Sharon adds:

> I never have had, and still don't have, the maternal feelings for her that I have for my other kids. We're good friends and I so love her, but it's like we're sisters. I wish she could have had a more normal life.[37]

Different again was the experience reported by Kathleen DeZeeuw, a rape victim who did experience maternal feelings, both before birth and in bringing up her child.[38] While she has a close relationship with her son to this day, the emotional effects of the rape, her later alcohol and drug abuse and her son's external resemblances to the rapist made for a turbulent and even violent upbringing for him. Kathleen has warm words of praise for her son, regrets what she put him through while he was growing up, and urges women in her situation to think carefully about the possibility of adoption, for the sake of the child. Kathleen does not, however, regret her own raising of—much less her giving birth to—the son she deeply loves. On the contrary, "The life I tried to snuff out was the very tool that was used to bring me to a place where I could forgive those involved in what happened to me." [39]

On the subject of abortion, which she herself attempted when she first found she was pregnant, Kathleen says:

> I believe that to encourage a woman to have an abortion is to add even more violence to her life. The fact that she is still alive should give her an added reason to cherish the innocent life growing inside her as well. Two wrongs will never make a right.[40]

CHILDBIRTH AND CHILDCARE

When considering the very real possibility that a woman will wish to raise a child conceived by rape, we need to bear in mind that in some environments, especially in the absence of a supportive family, there may be little chance that others will step in and look after the baby if one will not do so oneself. Caring for the baby in such a situation may be essential not just to the child's welfare but to his or her very survival. While admittedly, this may also be true of abandoned orphans, it takes a person of unusual detachment to see the baby one has just given birth to—even a child conceived by violence—as having no greater claim on one than a child found by the roadside. Of course, one might try to do one's best for either baby, but perhaps only one child can be fed or carried to safety: the first baby does seem to have a prior claim on what is surely its *mother*, however she became so. And in any event, whatever one's duty of positive support, to *kill* the child conceived by rape, simply for being so conceived, is surely not an option if the child like any other is a full, 'personal' moral subject.

Just as parental wanting or unwanting cannot change a baby's nature or its status, it cannot change the birth mother's (or father's) parental link with the baby,[41] though social aspects of this relationship may of course be delegated in some situations. Adoption may sometimes be the best solution for everyone, but it comes at a cost to both the birth mother and the child: for the mother (or birth parents), the adoption may be a source of life-long suffering,[42] and the child, even if adopted by very loving parents, loses a valuable connection to the person who not only provided months of nurture but who nearly always helped to cause the child's existence, and thus contributed to his or her makeup in more obvious ways. Knowing one's origins is important, as the efforts of adopted and now, donor-conceived people to access their biological parents would appear to demonstrate. And even where birth parents have every reason to believe that adoption is the best choice, both for them and for their child, adoption cannot cancel their duties entirely: these may reappear in unforeseen ways.[43] For example, it will often be right for birth parents to agree to meet the child in later life, if he or she makes contact.

To return to chosen parenthood: In the case of men, we certainly do *not* accept 'not feeling paternal' or not having chosen fatherhood as a reason for the man not to support his child, whether financially or in other ways. With the exception of cases of sperm donation—where the offspring themselves will sometimes insist on the parental tie—men are not, nor should they be, permitted to deny their paternity, merely on the basis that they did not choose to be fathers, understood as such.[44] There is, admittedly, a certain train of thought according to which childbirth and childrearing are lifestyle choices[45] to be indulged in at women's own discretion—but also at their own expense.[46] Already some commentators are challenging what they see as an injustice, and protesting that, if women can choose parenthood during pregnancy, parenthood should not be imposed on the man who did not choose it in any way.[47] With the 'choice' model of parenthood, which sees motherhood as arising not from (in most cases) chosen intercourse, but from chosen (continued) pregnancy,[48] motherhood by choice becomes fatherhood by choice as men lose duties to their own unchosen children. Women lose the support of men in raising children, with all that means emotionally and financially, and children lose the caring, adult input of the other person who—deliberately or otherwise—helped bring them into being.

With duties to act paternally towards a child come, however, rights—just as with maternal duties. If a man is morally obliged to support his child financially,[49] then (cases of abuse or incapacity aside) he is also obliged to support his child in psychological ways. That is his moral right, as well as his duty; nor should his wish to protect his child, including prenatally,[50] be seen as an intrusion: he also has nurturing duties towards the baby, even at this stage. Though the woman is surely the first guardian of the pregnancy, the man too has a clear parental stake in their child's welfare: those men who show their sense of this (as many sadly do not)[51] should be affirmed in so doing. It is neither logical nor psychologically realistic to tell either parent to put his or her sense of parental responsibility on hold until the other parent gives permission to express it. To reduce parenthood to *de facto* feelings of bonding is to fail to see that people can be better or worse parents in this as in other ways. At the same time, it is possible for either parent to resolve to be the best parent they can be, given that a parent is what they are. Far from *creating* the moral right and duty, bonding is *appropriate* to an existing relationship—though emotional aspects of that relationship can certainly take time to form, and are not entirely in one's control.

PREGNANCY AND CONTROL

Apart from a *prima facie* right and duty to raise the child—which the birth mother, birth father, or ideally both will have— what might be some other rights and duties of the parents and others during pregnancy itself? Before exploring this question, it may be worth taking a brief look at the experience of feeling 'out of control' during pregnancy: an experience women often report, despite the many processes their bodies are controlling.[52] One woman comments:

> Feelings of fear and anxiety consumed me, and I wasn't completely comfortable sharing them since they often seemed irrational. A life was growing inside me and I couldn't see it, feel it, or do anything to ensure its well-being. I never felt so out of control.[53]

Amy Mullin, who cites this comment, does not dismiss in any way such feelings of distress, or the other burdens pregnancy may bring, whether or not societally caused. Nonetheless, Mullin reflects as follows on her own experience of several very difficult and burdensome pregnancies:

> My own experiences with pregnancy taught me many things, and although I am relieved that they are over, I am grateful for more than the three children that resulted. The changes I experienced in pregnancy, including those changes relating to illness and impairment, were opportunities for me to learn what it is like to live with a body that had

become unreliable, that shifts and is uncanny, and that led me to experience vulnerability and dependence . . . pregnancy may . . . give practice in walking the balance between directing and accommodating change that continues once a pregnancy ends and, for some, when childrearing begins.[54]

In a similar vein, Brooke Shueneman comments that:

> In order to be pregnant and give birth, the mother must surrender some of the control of her body she once enjoyed. Compelled to allow her body to grow and change, surrendering becomes empowering. . . . She is able to escape from the pressures that tell her she must maintain a certain form and simply *be* as her body and her baby need her to be.[55]

In affluent societies much focused on physical appearance and the pursuit of chosen goals in work and recreation, practice in accepting and adapting to new circumstances and a new, uncharted relationship may have value far beyond the area of pregnancy itself. And if this is true of standard, healthy pregnancies, it applies still more to those requiring onerous additional precautions to sustain. An example might be the requirement of bed rest for a pregnancy at very high risk of miscarriage: in its strictest form this additional requirement may demand great generosity and endurance, verging on the supererogatory for some women.[56] Women in this situation will, moreover, have serious claims to support from those around them—and this support too has value and meaning beyond its utility in meeting the woman's current needs.

PREGNANCY AND GUARDIANSHIP

There is a benign aspect to societal interest in pregnancy, at least where this takes a certain form. Julie Piering observes that:

> . . . there is a sense of unity and kinship surrounding the activity of childbirth, here conceived as an expansion of community. Any member of society, then, is legitimately interested in and concerned for the pregnant woman. Although the immediate familiarity strangers permit themselves with a woman's body can be disconcerting, in some respects this interest operates as an extension of the familial model and can likewise be comforting. . . . [57]

Piering expands:

> As members of a community, we are all private individuals and autonomous subjects with public bodies. The community calls on our bodies,

and we call on each other to support communal undertakings . . . The pregnant body is an especially celebrated and scrutinized public body for it is the sine qua non for the continuation of the community. There can be no community without new members, and nothing can remind us of the fragility and beauty of persons and the connections they make quite as well as births.[58]

Piering's points are well taken: pregnancy should not be over-individualised to the point of denying legitimate community interest in a community event. Having said that, many feminist writers, including Piering,[59] have drawn attention to forms of social surveillance and control of pregnant women which are offensive by any reasonable standard. Thus Anna Smajdor comments:

for expectant mothers, the fact of encompassing another life in their bodies often takes a serious toll on their autonomy. Pregnant women are routinely expected to subsume their appetites and desires into those that would be in keeping with the well-being of the fetus. Not only this, but their abilities and rights to make decisions about their medical care are at risk of being overridden in favor of the interests of the unborn child. Respect for one's bodily integrity, something that most men may take for granted at least in a medical setting, is by no means assured for women even in societies that pride themselves on concern for ethics and autonomy. Women are still sterilized against their will and undergo forced abortions and forced caesarians.[60]

Much of what Smajdor describes here is certainly deplorable, particularly the bringing to bear of physical constraints and even forcible invasions of the pregnant woman's body, whether to harm or even to benefit her baby. This is not to say that women do not have their own, very real responsibilities to safeguard both their children and themselves. After all, any woman who expects her pregnancy to continue—and this quite irrespective of her views on fetal status—will unavoidably have *some* responsibility to minimize harm, including harm the child may not consciously experience for many years. To say this is not, of course, to say that *only* the child's interests must be considered, much less that society may authorize forcible invasions of the woman to protect the child's interests—as opposed to *prohibiting* needless and harmful interventions, consensual or otherwise (for example, the administering by doctors of drugs like thalidomide or worse, RU486). We do not have police at the family dinner table ensuring the intake of healthy food by children.[61] And while postnatal child neglect,[62] as well as child abuse, is admittedly a criminal offence, there are special reasons before birth to respect the woman's guardianship of the child,[63] since the child can *only* be benefitted through her—at least in terms of his or her immediate health. Aggressive attempts to promote the child's welfare prenatally may deter some women from seeking prenatal care or (in the case of women struggling with drug or alcohol dependency) rehabilitation programs. Even more seriously, such attempts may entrench habits of thinking in which women's interests are pitted against those of their children, even in standard situations where no major conflict exists. Already, the availability of abortion—an option which focuses harmfully on, and does not merely affect, the fetus—creates a noxious and artificial climate for women in which they and their babies are seen as at least potential foes. Women are routinely invited by those about them, including health professionals, to end the pregnancy relationship or see it as tentative at best.[64] Surveillance and physical constraints on pregnant women may further alienate some women from their babies and drive some to abortion who might otherwise have bonded further with and kept their child. Given that the woman is, in fact, the rightful guardian and custodian of her pregnancy, the impetus should be to encourage her own sense of responsibility for the baby and for herself, and to make available social resources to women (including younger, poorer, and disabled mothers) who may need special help.

The child is inevitably in the pregnant woman's care in a way it is in no one else's—including the father's. She is not only the parent but the 'body parent'—the parent whose body completely surrounds the child. This immediately engages her own health interests, as well as her social interest in her baby's welfare, and makes sense of an approach where her own views on risks and benefits for the baby and herself take precedence even over those of the child's father.

That means, however, not that the pregnant woman has *fewer* responsibilities than other people, but that she has more. For example, if the woman and the baby's father are painting a bedroom with paint they suddenly discover to be toxic to unborn children, both will have some responsibility for downing brushes, but more responsibility will arguably fall on her. There will be many situations in which reasonable parents will need to adjust their behavior in some way, whether their child is born or unborn.[65] This does not mean that either parent should be expected to put the child's interests first on every occasion: parents of a toddler may sometimes feed her fast food (when other food might be healthier) and chat to their friends (when the toddler might prefer a push on the swing). Family life is a matter of harmonizing interests which inevitably conflict to some extent, and this process begins during pregnancy or even before the child is conceived.

Amy Mullin's comments on maternal-fetal conflicts during pregnancy are of interest here:

> [F]etuses do matter, but a fetus is never the only factor in a pregnancy that has moral significance, and we are bound to err when we frame questions about pregnancy by thinking of pregnant women and fetuses as adversaries. However, this is not because a pregnant woman and her fetus are one entity; it is possible for their well-being to be at odds. It is

instead because to think of them as adversaries is to suppose that fetal interests may be advanced only at some cost to pregnant women. This is both false as a matter of fact (for instance, better nutrition, shelter, and living conditions may advance the interests of both) and mistaken in its assumption that pregnant women are the only ones who can affect fetal well-being.[66]

These observations seem entirely reasonable, including Mullin's recognition that it is possible, though not as common as is sometimes suggested, for the interests of the pregnant woman and fetus to conflict. The concluding section of this chapter will be devoted to exploring some all too real, though rather uncommon, medical conflicts which can arise between the woman and her baby. Before that, however, we will look very briefly at the phenomenon of prenatal testing: an area where tests and even abortions are often presented, albeit with little basis, as beneficial to the woman and/or baby (and others, it is sometimes frankly suggested).[67]

PRENATAL TESTS

Prenatal tests of an invasive kind such as amniocentesis and chorionic villus sampling are a source of fetal (or maternal-fetal) risk that comes paradoxically with heavy societal endorsement. These tests are normally offered not to protect the woman's health or that of the fetus but to give the woman information on the health of the fetus—in most cases, so she can consider an abortion should a problem be found. This is often not made clear to the woman before the test or earlier screening: the woman may simply be accepting a procedure presented as routine, or else seeking to dispel anxieties that screening itself may have raised. Admittedly, some fetal conditions can be treated in utero, or special arrangements made to deliver the baby, but that is not the standard situation. Again, if it truly is the case that a baby does not change its moral status just by changing its location (from within to outside the womb), then to offer an abortion to avoid the birth of a child with, say, Down Syndrome will be no more defensible than offering infanticide of a newborn child with Down's. Indeed, it may in some ways be worse, as the act takes place within the woman's body itself: the place where the child's life would normally be nurtured, not taken, and through which the woman's physical health, as well as her psyche, may be harmed. The harrowing experience for the woman of such abortions, and the fact that the fetus is often referred to as a baby by women and medical staff alike,[68] would tend to support the view that the life here targeted is recognized to be that of a child. If Down Syndrome babies, like the rest of us, have lives and interests[69] that should be respected, this will apply throughout their lifespan, and not only for the postnatal period. The same can, indeed, be said of far more serious conditions,[70] including ones where the baby cannot long survive birth: if we cherish older dying people in their final days, often in a hospice-type environment, this should apply no less to babies who are dying, whose families similarly need help from those about them of a generous and well-informed kind. (The poignant situation of lethal anomaly, and the responses of some women who carry their babies to term, are explored briefly in an Appendix to this book.)

Some women experience difficulty declining tests during pregnancy which are oriented to a possible abortion: health professionals can be surprisingly insistent in proposing and re-proposing tests to women as 'prenatal care'.[71] This is particularly objectionable in the case of tests which carry a real risk of causing a miscarriage: one in 100 or 200 are figures still sometimes cited for chorionic villus sampling and amniocentesis. While even pregnant women who are unreservedly committed to their babies may nonetheless want to allay their fears, or else prepare for the birth of a disabled child, few parents would agree to a test of a *new*born child which had a one-in-a-hundred chance of killing that child and had no therapeutic purpose, but merely speeded up diagnosis. If the fetus is a child, no such test should be performed on it which is more dangerous than we would accept after birth, whether the child is able-bodied or disabled, healthy or terminally ill. Indeed, there is even *less* reason to take such risks if the child is still unborn, given that miscarriage is a physical, and not just a social, harm to the woman who loses her baby. It is ironic that a society which instructs pregnant women to avoid much lesser risks to themselves and their babies during pregnancy should regard these greater risks with such apparent equanimity.

MATERNAL AND MATERNAL-FETAL TREATMENTS

What can we say about situations in which either the fetus or the pregnant woman could derive genuine health benefit from, not a test, but a medical treatment foreseen to cause or risk serious harm to the other party? This area is difficult, in every sense of the word, and deserves exploring at some length. To focus on the most difficult cases, I will look not just at cases where treatment, though needing consent and posing risks, has a clear potential benefit to mother and baby, but at cases where one party alone is intended to benefit overall in terms of health, while the other will risk or incur serious harm. It is worth bearing in mind in what follows that probabilities of harm resulting from actions taken or not taken may be different for each party: for example, harm for one if action is taken may be more probable than harm for the other if nothing is done.

TREATMENTS IN PREGNANCY—CONJOINED TWIN ANALOGY

In the introduction to this book, we looked briefly at the case of conjoined twins—a sustained physical connection between two related human beings—as a possible analogy for pregnancy. Unlike with pregnancy, there is some clear sharing of parts with conjoined twins, while as with pregnancy, operations on one subject will not benefit the other's health in every situation. The analogy may therefore be helpful to bear in mind when considering maternal-fetal conflicts, not least because life-threatening conflicts, as well as less serious conflicts, can also arise with conjoined twins. While it is true that the relationship of twins is one of siblinghood and hence without the 'guardianship' dimension of pregnancy—a very important aspect of this archetypal mother-child bond—we can deal to some extent with this difference by imagining that one of a pair of (adult) conjoined twins is not only physically dependent on the other but mentally disabled, so reliant on the stronger twin to make decisions for both.

To begin with a more everyday scenario: in the case of drinking alcohol, it would appear that the stronger twin should give some consideration to the interests of the weaker, even if he may sometimes put his own interests first (he might, for example, have a glass of wine sometimes, despite the fact this will mildly impact the interests of his sibling—for example, keep him up at night). Often, though, the weaker twin will need to be deferred to, not least because he is unable to defend his own interests, and sometimes the sacrifices called for from the stronger twin will not be so minor.

For example, imagine that the weaker twin needs an operation on some part of his own body, in the course of which surgeons will need to put both twins under anesthetic, and perhaps even go through some part of the body of the stronger twin to access the body of the weaker. Unpleasant as this may be for the stronger twin to contemplate, depending on the level of his aversion and the risks and benefits involved, he might sometimes have a duty to accept it for the sake of his more vulnerable sibling. Perhaps the notion of duty may not even arise here, as the idea of refusing may seem unthinkable—but some natural shrinking from surgery may occur even in the most united of siblings, at which point some may find the thought of fraternal duty helpful.

Note, however, that doctors should not offer surgery which is too damaging to the interests of the stronger twin—for example, if he will never heal from it but will be seriously impaired. Nor should doctors, even with minor surgery, impose it on the stronger twin should he choose to refuse it: if we are talking about his own body, not his twin's, he would need to authorize invasions of that body even if those invasions were in his own health interests, as here they are not.

The same is true, mutatis mutandis, of maternal consent to maternal-fetal surgery, where in contrast, there is *never* any access to the more dependent and fragile person's body except through the body of the supporter. As in the conjoined twins case, the supporter here is entitled to ask searching questions about the probabilities: the woman is much less likely to have any duty to accept any treatment where the outcome is very uncertain, and the risks and burdens for her and/or the baby very high. In contrast, more standard procedures like fetal blood transfusions may well be procedures the woman should normally accept, and the doctor should strongly recommend—although certainly they may not be imposed.

Unlike the stronger conjoined twin, who may not benefit at all in terms of health from a healthy outcome for his sibling, the pregnant woman has, it seems, a 'reproductive health interest' in delivering a live and (if possible) healthy baby once the child has been conceived. Just as a woman is less healthy reproductively if she is carrying a gene that will endanger any child she conceives, she is less healthy reproductively if she cannot carry her actual child[72] to term. Promoting a safe and healthy birth for her baby is in her presumptive health interests, as well as her child's—though her 'reproductive health interest' in doing this[73] may, in some high-risk situations, be at odds with her general health interest in avoiding bodily harm.[74] (The woman will also, of course, have a moral/social interest in avoiding injustice to her child in any choices she may make. Our physical flourishing is of real value, and some of our rights do concern that flourishing, but respect for others and ourselves must be maintained while our health is pursued.)

DUTIES TO COMMENCE GESTATION

Might a woman sometimes have a duty to become pregnant in the first place if her embryos already exist—for example, if she has had 'spare' embryos frozen after IVF? Here the likelihood of benefiting any given embryo may not be high, as many frozen embryos die when thawed, or do not go to term. However, one might argue that one is obliged to 'go the extra mile' if one is responsible, in some strong sense, for the plight of a dependent child—assuming this is what the embryo is. The fact that there are embryos in need of 'rescue' from the freezer is wholly due to their production in vitro in greater numbers than can be immediately transferred to the body of the genetic mother. So 'treatment' for both the woman and the embryos, in the form of transfer of the embryos to her body, might well be morally required if it is medically straightforward.[75] It does, however, seem that the morality of *commencing* gestation is different from the morality of *continuing* gestation: in the second case, though not the first, issues of bodily invasion of the child and other issues of 'positive harm'—as opposed to failure to aid —can arise. That said, a woman who failed to have her embryos transferred with the *intention* that they die would act similarly in moral terms to someone who deliberately sought the same result by other means.

CONJOINED TWINS CONTINUED

To return briefly to the conjoined twins analogy: what if, in contrast, the stronger or more able twin himself needs medical treatment which will be harmful—perhaps even fatal—to his sibling, but does not itself target the sibling's body in any way? Perhaps in this case the stronger/more able twin is, again, morally entitled to accept treatment, at least if the sibling is already close to death. Harm to the twin, like other effects on the twin's body, is here a (serious) side-effect of treatment, not something purposely sought. Such side-effects in or outside medicine may sometimes be accepted: for example, the rescuer who closes a fire door, foreseeing that those trapped behind will be lethally affected, may well be justified if no deaths are intended, and if other lives will be saved.[76] We will say more about side-effects shortly.

Similar, if not identical, things can be said about a woman who needs medical treatment for her own body and whose baby will be killed, or at least risk death, if the treatment is performed.[77] For example, a woman might need urgent cancer treatment: while risks to the baby can often be minimized, and many cancer treatments are not especially risky,[78] treatment such as hysterectomy will certainly kill a pre-viable baby, but may still be urgently required to save the mother's life.[79] Note, however, that deliberate removal—let alone deliberate bodily invasion of the baby—is not the issue here: the very same treatment would be required if the woman were not currently pregnant.

Now consider a case in which, in contrast, the weaker or less able con-joined twin is himself endangering his sibling, such that lethal invasions of the weaker twin's own body would be needed to save the stronger/more able twin. Should we carry out such lethal invasions on the weaker twin—the unwitting source of the threat? Many would say yes, but that answer may be too quick: would such interventions violate respect for the weaker twin's own bodily borders, and thereby for the twin himself? Would we stop the heart of the weaker twin deliberately, if that would benefit the other? Mutilate him? Reallocate his organs? [80]

VITAL CONFLICTS: WHAT ARE THE PRINCIPLES?

At this point, a pause may be in order to think about these conflicts, which can arise both in and outside medicine, in a more systematic way.[81] One approach to conflict situations is to see the individual who creates the threat, however unwittingly, as an aggressor who may therefore be deliberately harmed (including lethally) or at least made the object of deliberate bodily invasions of a harmful kind—of which more below. However, such an approach to 'material,' unintended threats, at least, is really very questionable. That becomes easier to see if we imagine that each party is threatening the other—say, because they are both breathing air while they are trapped in a confined space where the oxygen is running out. (This case might correspond to a case of obstructed labor in which the woman and her baby are effectively threatening each other: the baby's presence is dan-gerous to the woman if her contractions cannot cause delivery, while these contractions are also dangerous to the baby.) Would each person in the confined space be entitled to attack the other purposely—say, by strangulation or by clamping the other's mouth—to defend himself against the other's *un*intentional threat of oxygen deprivation? That does not seem reasonable: more is surely required than sheer coexistence and breathing of air to justify such an assault.[82]

Moreover, even if endangerment goes only one way—from a person needing some resource to a person supplying that resource—there seems to be a difference between endangerment which is, in every sense, unwitting and endangerment which results at least from an act deliberately directed at the endangered person (or at something he or she is known to possess). It is one thing to respond to endangerment of the second kind by deliberately attacking/invading someone who is non-culpably trying to injure or make (fatal) use of me: an insane person, say, or someone frantically trying to climb on top of me as we both struggle in deep water. It is something quite different to attack or invade someone who is trying to do no such thing— and who has, moreover, no intentions whatever in my regard, whether to use my body as a useful floating object (although this will drown me) or to use it as a source of oxygen (although this will kill me by making my heart 'work for two'). If someone has no plans in my (or others') regard, that person is surely innocent[83] in the full sense of the term. To deny this would, moreover, yield a highly counterintuitive result in a case in which it is the woman who is endangering her viable baby by remaining pregnant (say, when she is very close to death). Could such a woman really be seen as an 'aggressor', such that *anything* we need to do to rescue her baby, whatever that means for her, would be morally justified? Is she not rather a 'fellow-victim' with the baby of a situation neither has caused in any sense that justifies a violent response?

DOUBLE-EFFECT REASONING

Many of those who accept that the woman and her baby do have equal moral status see these questions simply in terms of whether death or bodily harm is *intended*, and then in terms of whether it is *unfair* to cause such harm as an unintended side-effect. Intentions are, indeed, very important in ethics: they help define what we are doing. There is all the difference in the world between doing high-risk surgery on cancer patients in the awareness that some will 'die on the table', and doing the same procedures, as perhaps a Nazi doctor might do them, with the *intention* that some die. Our moral decisions, whether serious or trivial, will often make use of 'double-effect reasoning' according to which merely foreseen aspects of these decisions are evaluated differently from aspects we intend. That is the reason why, on this approach, the woman who accepts a cancer treatment that harms her unborn child can be justified: neither death nor harm is intended, as an end or means, while what the woman *does* intend—a healing invasion of her body alone—is in itself a good intention. To go through the traditional steps of double-effect reasoning (or at least, one formulation of these steps), the immediate act is good, the harm is not intended, the good is not achieved via the harm, and there is due proportion between the good and bad effects, assuming the woman has a good chance of being cured.

'UNINTENDED MORALLY DETERMINATIVE ASPECTS'[84]

However, it is important to remember (and is often forgotten in double-effect discussions) that an intention *to kill or harm as such* is not the only bad intention to look out for. An intention *to invade or affect the body* of an innocent person, as an end or means, in a way we *know* is seriously harmful is another bad intention which, I want to claim, is *also* morally conclusive. Certain intentions, along with certain foreseen harms, are *jointly* conclusive, such that not all side-effects are 'mere' side-effects which could, in principle, be outweighed by sufficiently good intended effects.[85] If I intend to harvest your heart while you are still alive, any truth in my claim (an empirical claim about my mental state) that I do not intend to kill you, but 'merely' to take your heart, cannot suffice to make my action right. The space your body fills, like my own body-space, must be respected and must not be lethally invaded, since you are an innocent fellow human being with no plans to affect me in any way.

Am I saying that, in this case, there is at least an *intention to harm* the person I invade? Not necessarily: if I lack the intention to cause death in performing a deliberate (and lethal) bodily invasion, I may equally lack the intention to cause injury—which similarly may not advance my goals, or be imagined to advance them. Nonetheless, it is surely enough that the *invasion itself* is intended, and that a lethal effect, and no therapeutic effect, on my victim is foreseen. What makes the action wrong, I am claiming, is that the intention to invade the victim's body is coupled with the foresight that this will not promote, [86] but will instead seriously harm, the bodily functioning of that person. Nor is the victim's proximity to death relevant: lethal organ harvesting violates justice in violating the victim's bodily borders, even if the victim has only hours or minutes to live. This also holds, I would argue, even if, through no choice or wish of the victim's own, the victim is posing a lethal threat to some other human being.

It is possible to describe unintended features of our actions, such as that their target is alive, innocent and vulnerable,[87] as a 'circumstance' of those actions. However, such features should really be given another term (see this section heading for one suggestion) as they necessarily enter into the moral description of the act, in conjunction with what we *do* intend.[88] We can think of the case mentioned in the previous chapter, where I am trapped under the body of someone—we can even imagine, a close family member—in a way that threatens to cause me harm. Cutting into someone who is alive (and innocent) and who is known to be alive (and innocent) is quite a different act from cutting into someone dead. This is so even if such cutting has the same immediate intention—clearing away the bodily obstruction—and the same further intention—saving life. There may be nothing wrong with *some* cuttings-up of bodies, but the 'circumstance' that the 'body' in front of me is alive—the living body of an innocent human being—is not a *mere* circumstance, even if my intentions focus only on cutting away what is before me. The bodily rights of human beings do not lapse just because they are already facing death—or even because the body of the dying person threatens that of someone else. Those who intend no effect at all on others but are mere 'hapless bystanders' to the threat their bodies pose are in fact non-aggressors, and should not be subjected to deliberate bodily invasions of this kind.

BODILY RESPECT

Respect for a person includes respect for that person's bodily borders. We need to remember that (as we saw in the first chapter) human persons are bodily beings, whose rights and interests, assuming they have rights and interests, will involve their own bodily 'space'. In a world where it is unreasonable to expect all harmful impact on others of our actions to be avoided—we do, after all, share 'space' in the sense of what surrounds us—it is perfectly possible and reasonable to expect everyone to respect each other's bodily space, in the sense that we do not deliberately invade the space of others in what we know are harmful ways. Even 'shovings' or other harmful movings need at least to be justified in some way—but something much stronger can be said of seriously harmful incursions on someone's personal space *while the person occupies that space*. Fair negotiation of 'common space' between human beings gives no title to such bodily incursions. Whatever the other bodily rights of innocent human beings, any rights they have surely include the right not to have others 'take it upon themselves' to invade their bodies in ways that do not benefit their health but do them serious permanent harm.

MATERNAL-FETAL CONFLICTS CONTINUED

To return to pregnancy: there are additional sources of complexity here which do not arise with conjoined twins—let alone with other, less intimate bodily connections. To begin with, in pregnancy the body of one subject is entirely contained within the body of the other, which means that anyone attempting to justify an intervention to benefit the fetus will *always* need to justify an intervention on the woman, since her body will always be invaded. And sometimes, the effects on her will simply be too harmful, as when a dying woman might be invaded to rescue her viable fetus in a way which does her serious permanent harm (we can imagine a procedure—perhaps a crude procedure outside a normal hospital environment[89]—which will immediately kill a woman who is so gravely ill that she will not recover from it).[90] Even if a competent woman requested the procedure to save her baby's life, it is hard to see how health professionals could be justified in such a harmful incursion on a patient, even to save a second patient in their care.[91] Others may judge such cases differently, but this would be, I think, a very dubious thing for the woman to request, however generous her motive. It is rather as if she were to volunteer herself for lethal experimentation or lethal organ harvesting: the bodily self of human beings is not property—not even of the human being herself. To say that a patient has first responsibility for her own health is not to say that she may authorize all and any interventions she wishes but rather that she may *veto* even healing interventions she judges inappropriate, as she is the normal source of the doctor's authority to act.[92] 'Charity begins at home' and the right to basic bodily respect and non-mutilation cannot be waived. We should respect our own bodies, as well as those of other innocent people, when it comes to gravely harmful bodily invasions.

In contrast, when we are treating the woman's body alone, in her own interests, as with, say, hysterectomy for cancer, 'vital conflicts' will be easier to deal with, though great sadness may remain. Admittedly, side-effects for the baby must be considered, but even lethal side-effects may surely be accepted if the woman's own chance of benefiting is high—and even if not one but two babies will be lost.[93] It is, after all, the woman's body, not that of the baby or babies that is targeted here. Moreover—and this may be conclusive—because the baby or babies are still entirely surrounded by the woman's body, even the side-effects take place uniquely within the outer (and the inner) borders of another human being. The space affected, albeit unintentionally, is the baby or babies' own body-space—which, however, is still within the woman's special 'sphere of influence.' For that reason, such side-effects appear more tolerable morally than side-effects for someone located entirely outside her body—say, a breastfeeding baby. This may be one difference from the conjoined twins case, where causing lethal injury to a twin who is *not* already dying—even if that twin's body is in no way targeted—is more difficult to justify, involving as it does positive harm and the reversal of each twin's chance of long-term survival.

It might help to think of a country which contains another country completely within its own borders: such a country might be thought to have a special relationship with that smaller country, involving, on the one hand, a particular duty to offer aid when necessary and, on the other, a more permissive approach when urgent interventions on the larger country (say, use of a dangerous insecticide to combat some environmental disaster) would harmfully impact the smaller country. Alternatively, we might think of harms internal to a household: if a very poor family in a developing country is forced to use dangerous chemicals in their home-based work, which are lethally affecting the grandmother's health, the fact that she is already intimately involved in the family fortunes as a live-in family member may mean it is permissible in extremis to cause these lethal side-effects for her, while it would not be permissible to cause them to the grandmother next door.

LIFE-THREATENING PREGNANCIES

As always with pregnancy, analogies limp, though and for the rest of the chapter we will not depart more than momentarily from pregnancy itself.

Whatever we think about cases in which no effect at all is intended for the party who is lethally harmed, the really difficult cases of maternal-fetal conflict arise when it is pregnancy specifically, not some parallel condition such as cancer, which is endangering the woman's life. Examples might be pulmonary hypertension, in which pregnancy increases the woman's risk of heart failure, or ectopic pregnancy, in which the embryo implants outside the woman's womb and can endanger her life if it continues to grow.

How should we respond to these very real instances of maternal-fetal 'conflict' in the very strongest sense, while fully respecting both lives affected and the unique bond they share? We will begin with cases where the treatment method proposed involves a bodily invasion of the fetus itself, and then look at cases where no bodily invasion, but nonetheless deliberate removal and/or detachment from the mother is involved.

In fact, deliberate removal or detachment, whether done surgically or 'at one remove' by administering a drug, will in practice very often involve a harmful invasion of fetal tissues, including the amniotic sac and other fetal membranes, in the course of extracting the fetus from the mother. To return to the themes of the introduction: we should not see the unborn child as a mere miniature adult shape. This is no more appropriate for the fetus than for the early embryo; nor is there any reason to see (for example) the fetal placenta as anything other than an organ of the fetus, albeit one discarded at birth. While the fetus is of course functionally dependent both on the fetal placenta and on the very much smaller maternal placenta, only the first is produced by the baby and normally genetically the same as the so-called 'fetus proper'. Nor can the fact it is discarded at birth retrospectively make the fetal placenta not part of the baby; after all, on similar reasoning, the maternal placenta would not be part of the mother (and of course other parts like the milk teeth are discarded during childhood).

In view of all this, to speak of 'mere removal' or 'mere detachment' from the mother pre-viability may be unrealistic. With the possible exception of interventions that prevent implantation, or hypothetically target, not the fetal placental or other tissues, but only the smaller maternal placenta,[94] in speaking of separation pre-viability we will often be speaking about a deliberate (and effectively lethal) invasion of the child's own bodily borders—even if the invasion is sought as a mere means to benefit the mother, and the lethal effect is not sought at all. If it is indeed wrong (as suggested above) to invade lethally the body of a pregnant woman, even a dying woman, to rescue her viable child, how can it be right to invade lethally the body of an unborn child to rescue her mother?

To return to 'aggression': it may be claimed that, however innocently, the fetal or embryonic child is in fact endangering her mother in this life-threatening situation, and so can be treated as an aggressor such that her own body may now be invaded. To repeat: one problem with this move—apart from the oddity of terms like 'aggressor'[95] when no threat is intended—is that it could equally be applied to the dying woman who is pregnant with a viable baby: her body may be 'trapping' the baby she supports, who would now be very much safer outside it, but this does not deprive the woman of her right to bodily immunity. This is surely the case whether the woman is competent to make her own decisions or has—perhaps permanently—lost that capacity, such that others must make decisions for her. Always assuming that mother and child equally have strong rights, as innocent human beings, not to have their bodies harmfully invaded, we will need to negotiate our way through these situations with considerably more care.

ECTOPIC PREGNANCY

The case of tubal ectopic pregnancy, the most common form of ectopic (i.e., out of place)[96] pregnancy, can present a range of scenarios, not all of which pose especially serious ethical problems. To begin with, there is the unproblematic practice of 'expectant management' of an ectopic pregnancy which is discovered early and which poses no immediate threat. Expectant management is sometimes proposed not for the sake of the embryo but for the sake of the woman, to spare her what may well be unnecessary treatment in particular situations. Many early ectopics miscarry naturally before an emergency is reached, and doctors will sometimes recommend 'watchful waiting', rather than drug treatment (discussed below) to see if this occurs.

Should the pregnancy *not* miscarry, however, and should the tube be damaged by the embryo, the option may arise of removing the damaged tube, with the embryo still inside it. Unfortunately, such removal may impact the woman's fertility, although normally such impact will not be significant,[97] bearing in mind that many women will be left with one remaining functioning tube. However, in emergency situations, tube removal may now be the only reasonable option, even if the embryo, albeit close to death, is still alive (at least before any clamping of the woman's blood vessels, which will inevitably cut off the embryo's oxygen supply). This seems very similar to the case of removing a cancerous uterus, except that the unborn child is historically the cause of the damage to the woman's body-part—which would, however, need to be removed at this point, even if the embryo had already miscarried. No attack on the life, the body or even the presence of the embryo in the pregnant woman need be intended: here, the soon-to-die embryo has caused what is now an independent threat.

More difficult to defend are treatment methods in which the embryo or fetus itself, including fetal membranes like the trophoblast/placenta,[98] is deliberately targeted while the embryo is still alive.[99] This can be done either by opening up the tube and directly removing while—in practice[100]—harmfully invading the embryo (for example, using pressurized irrigation or forceps) or else by targeting the embryo and its own tissues at an earlier stage, using the drug methotrexate (MTX), which attacks rapidly dividing cells. Here the intention is not only to invade the trophoblast but to thwart its functioning in searching for nutrients—embryonic functioning which endangers the mother, taking place as it does in entirely the wrong environment since the tube cannot support long-term growth.[101] Destroying the embryonic trophoblast/placenta is, however, no less lethal mutilation than cutting the windpipe of a newborn baby—let's say, to prevent it breathing air which others need and which cannot long support it. The fact that the baby might have survived with a windpipe transplant, or the fetus with a futuristic artificial womb-with-placenta, is not relevant here, any more than normal hospital cesarians are relevant to the cutting open of pregnant women in circumstances in which they will certainly die. Whether an intended bodily invasion does serious harm,[102] and would harm even a healthy individual of the relevant age,[103] is what is morally conclusive here—or so I am proposing. The body-space of an innocent human being cannot be treated as just another part of the world or invaded if this will serve the interests of another—albeit also innocent and threatened by the presence of the first.

Finally, there is the option of taking out the tube, or the affected segment of the tube, not because it is already so damaged as to justify removal in any case, but to preempt further damage by the embryo, whose removal with the tube is here purposely achieved. Just as with uterine cancer, the womb is standardly removed as a means of removing the cancerous cells inside it, here the tube is removed precisely as containing, not a cancer but an embryo who may cause future harm, before or after its future death. To many, such intentional removal of the embryo (with a relatively undamaged tube) seems clearly justifiable in principle, and arguments against it seem well-nigh incomprehensible, in view of the risks this could avoid. And yet, an argument could be run that, in removing the child deliberately—even when its body-space is not deliberately invaded—a line is crossed that is not crossed either with expectant management, or with removal of an already-damaged tube.

This line is the unconditional commitment of the pregnant woman to her baby: 'till death [or birth] us do part'.[104] Perhaps there is some value in the mother-child relationship beginning at least, however it matures, in this starkly unconditional way. If so, then pregnancy would be, once again, a special case: the duty not to evict or withdraw support deliberately, at least before the baby is viable, would be, uniquely, absolute. Such unconditionality would enable pregnant women quite generally to bond especially closely with the children they are carrying, whose lives are accepted by their mothers as inextricably bound up with their own. While later on, parenthood is a matter of gradual 'letting go', introduction to other carers, and encouragement to independence, perhaps it is important that both mother and child feel that there was one time, at least, at which the child was supported literally unconditionally. Pregnancy would then involve a particularly generous commitment to the baby, whose presence is accepted as a 'given': any deliberate removal of the child pre-viability, or willingness to do so in certain circumstances, would cut against that primal commitment. Quite generally, ethics is more about 'input' than 'output'; more about attitudes than just about results: that, at least, is the best way of making sense of some of our own attitudes and feelings. As J.L.A. Garcia has argued,[105] we do not simply want other people to *affect* us in good ways, but to have good attitudes towards us. Many of us feel this way intuitively, whatever moral theory we may espouse. And such good attitudes may be especially important with the original, archetypal bond that is pregnancy: the bond between a mother and her child at the very start while their bodies are still very tightly connected.[106]

It may seem to be straining things unconscionably to apply such a view to a case in which the baby is lodged in the tube, where no baby ought to be (except, of course, appropriately en route to the womb). The tube may be the baby's 'home' in effect—but a highly temporary, precarious home, and not one functionally geared in any way to its shelter and protection at this stage. However, in uterine pregnancy too, the child can be 'misplaced' (where the placenta covers the opening to the cervix), and, if these considerations are to count, it may be difficult to draw clear lines with regard to deliberate removals, whether or not the child's body is invaded.[107] Be that as it may, concerns about deliberate removals, often accompanied by religious considerations, do, in fact, prevent some women from accepting, and some doctors from offering, this kind of targeting of embryos. Other options will be chosen, such as removing the tube should its own damaged state require this, if expectant management (for pregnancies discovered early) is not followed by miscarriage.

What is at stake, here and elsewhere, is not 'only' a life, or lives, but a relationship.[108] This is perhaps easiest to see in the case of what are very clearly bodily invasions. Just as cutting through a dying pregnant woman in such a way as to kill her immediately would be relationally a disrespectful act—however little the woman's life was in fact shortened—the same is true of the ectopic embryo cut into or otherwise invaded in an attempt to spare the mother's tube and thus her reproductive health.[109] In other words, we owe our fellow human beings, where they are innocent of crime or plans to harm us, respect for their bodily borders, so that justice is inevitably engaged when those borders are harmfully infringed. If painful conflicts can occur between adults, where bodily respect for an innocent fellow human being demands a costly forbearance, there is no reason to presume that such conflicts cannot arise in obstetric care—where the issue of deliberate removal as well as bodily invasions will come into play. That said, in modern obstetrics, threats to life itself can almost always be averted for the woman without recourse to deliberate attacks on the body or the presence of her child.

EARLY DELIVERY

Post-viability 'removals' are, of course, another matter, though serious ethical problems can arise here too in cases of extreme prematurity, where delivery brings a high probability of killing a child not otherwise in danger—or for whom delivery will greatly increase, rather than diminish, the danger. We need to distinguish between gestation itself—which is often basic care, and is never medical treatment—and other measures which may be necessary to bring a high-risk pregnancy to term or to a safer stage.

Some writers have spoken of bringing a pregnancy to term (including in cases in which the baby is already dying) as if the woman's simply remaining pregnant could—where there is a "substantive maternal risk"—constitute "active medical intervention on behalf of the fetus."[110] If refraining from delivery, rather than actively seeking to prolong the pregnancy,[111] is really what is meant here, this view seems strained given the basic, functional nature of the maternal-fetal connection, coupled with the bodily invasion of both mother and child involved in severing that connection. (Again, we need to remember that what are sometimes called the 'fetal tissues' are indeed precisely that: the amniotic sac and fetal placenta are organs grown by the fetus, not the mother.)[112] In contrast, hospitalization, medicine and surgery will be more often beyond the call of duty, particularly in cases where the baby has such serious anomalies that it cannot long survive. Early delivery, however, as involving active, hazardous moving of the child, however achieved, and disruption of its own tissues, must be evaluated more strictly, even if the child has a lethal anomaly and/or viability has (at least technically) been reached.[113] If the child will not itself benefit from early delivery in terms of health, then causing a high risk of death or serious bodily harm by delivering right on viability seems difficult to justify, especially for a psychological indication. In any case, it is difficult to show a psychological benefit to the mother from such an early delivery: even the grief of losing her baby—a great social harm, if not a medical harm—seems in practice to be easier to deal with and recover from when the woman takes her child to term.[114] Operative here is likely to be the feeling of the woman that she was 'there' for the baby as long as it needed her: their link was respected not just before, but even after, the point where healthy babies, if sadly not her own baby, have at least a fighting chance.[115]

NOTES

1 Anca Gheaus speaks eloquently of the value and likelihood of maternal bonding in pregnancy, although she does not recognize the moral, as opposed to legal (452), rights of parents that can surely exist prior to such bonding and make it appropriate, just as bonding can then reinforce rights:
   "I assume that intimate relationships are intrinsically valuable for those who are involved in them and that the incipience of such relationships during most pregnancies is to some extent unavoidable, given the bodily connection between fetus and gestating mother. It would therefore be both undesirable and very difficult, if possible, to prevent the formation of parent-baby relationships during gestations" (Anca Gheaus, "The Right to Parent One's Biological Baby", *Journal of Political Philosophy* 20.4 [2012]: 436).

2 Of course, most women—even those seeking to conceive—will not be conscious of their pregnancy at the outset, and any pregnancy will involve unconsciousness in the form of sleep.

3 The fact that rape, whatever the woman's degree of awareness, and whether or not it causes physical injury, is a serious 'offense against the person' is a sign not only of our bodily nature as persons, but of the fact that sex (and conception and gestation) are in some way 'special' (see Pruss, *One Body*, 70–76).

4 The continuing pregnancy can be seen as part of the injustice of the rapist's act, which, like so many other parts of that injustice, simply cannot be undone. Thus Mary Geach suggests that the rapist who makes a 10-year-old girl pregnant deprives her in so doing of the very right not to gestate (Mary Geach, "Motherhood, IVF and Sexual Ethics", in *Fertility and Gender*, ed. Helen Watt [Oxford: Anscombe Bioethics Centre, 2011], 175). Whatever our views on abortion following rape, we would surely have to say something rather like this about care of the rape-conceived newborn should the 10-year old girl be left with no one to assist her when the baby is born. She had, at one time, a (non-absolute) right not to be sole carer of a child, as she is only a child herself, but has been wrongly deprived of that right by an act of violence thanks to which her newborn needs her to survive.

5 I am excluding a hypothetical case where a doctor might 'remake' a woman pregnant by transferring her ectopic embryo to her womb in the interests of both her and the embryo (see note 100 of this chapter).

6 Boonin, *Defense of Abortion*, 166–7.

7 Rosalie Ber, "Ethical Issues in Gestational Surrogacy", *Theoretical Medicine* 21 (2000): 165, 167. The offence here is in making—as opposed to keeping—the unconscious woman pregnant with a genetically unrelated embryo. Here too, once pregnant, the woman would have a real maternal role and maternal rights, albeit wrongfully created: should she wake up and wish to keep the baby after birth, she should be permitted to do so as should any 'surrogate' mother, as I argue below.

8 On the issue of deliberate abortion in such cases, Beckwith comments:
   "It is hard to imagine that any doctor, in good conscience, would perform an abortion on this woman merely because he had no evidence that she had consented to the pregnancy. It is likely that those who had undergone such an abortion would experience a tragic sense of loss; a sense of having been robbed of something precious in the pregnancy—something which, at the very least, deserved thoughtful consideration despite the difficulties of bearing a child. It is hard to imagine that a woman in such circumstances would not herself feel significantly violated. In other words . . . the abortion, not the pregnancy, would be more analogous to rape" (Beckwith, *Defending Life*, 177).

9   For an argument that brain-damaged pregnant women, even if still alive (some are diagnosed, rightly or wrongly, as already dead) should not be assisted to support their pregnancies by technological means, see Nelson, "The Architect and the Bee". Despite the author's strong objections to 'unconscious pregnancy' (she explicitly extends her argument on cadaveric pregnancy to pregnancy in comatose women), she does accept that a woman might be supported technologically for a few weeks at the very end of pregnancy, as an alternative to her baby being born premature and having to receive (say) a week's intensive care (266). However, if it truly were demeaning and tantamount to rape to support a comatose woman for the sake of her pregnancy, even brief support of her for such a purpose would surely be morally excluded.

Nelson does make some valid points about the financial cost of such technological support: the money might indeed be better spent elsewhere. Less palatable is her suggestion that support might be withheld, not as disproportionately costly, but because the woman might not have wanted her baby to survive and 'burden' the father with his or her care (253). The implication here is that this would be a reasonable preference; however, a preference that one's baby not survive would surely not be a good reason for refusing consent to life-support, nor should we too quickly assume of any woman that she 'would take' this attitude to such an extraordinary situation.

10   This right, as I see it, is a 'human' right: the woman's absolute negative right not to be (here, non-consensually) aborted.

11   Belief that abortion is morally wrong can certainly coexist with a very unenthusiastic view of pregnancy itself, as Christopher Coope points out (*Worth and Welfare*, 14–15). However, this belief is surely more naturally coupled with a willing and generous (if also practical and unsentimental) 'welcoming' of the new life. Coope is perhaps overstating it when he says:

"The mistaken idea that the objection to abortion has something to do with an odd enthusiasm for birth—perhaps it will be called 'pro-natalism'—is very common. Yet why must someone opposed to abortion (or indeed contraception, since that seems also to be under discussion) think that a woman ought always to welcome being pregnant? . . . A woman might well be heard to say: '*Dammit, I'm pregnant again!*' How could anyone take exception to that? It would be quite in line for a friend who takes it for granted that an abortion would be murder to sympathise with her: '*Rotten luck!*' Perhaps the woman is determined this time *not* to fall in with 'the vision of a woman's role'. She will have the child adopted. Far from protesting, opponents of abortion might well be offering to assist her" (Coope, 14–15).

One does not have to pretend that pregnancy, childbirth and childrearing are light burdens in order to recognize one's maternal role and willingly 'step up to the plate' where it is possible and reasonable to do so. To say this is not, of course, to deny the very real responsibilities of others, beginning with the father of the child.

12   The pregnant woman is still 'holding' the baby—rather like a birth mother who may have promised to adopt out her child but is still in practice caring for it.

13   Nor does the situation seem different when the child has not yet been conceived: it is difficult to see why we should think that, in Andrea Stumpf's words, "existence begins in the minds of the desiring parents" (195–6) or that 'desiring motherhood' (I would say, would-be motherhood) has been "obfuscated" by the biological reality of gestation:

"The psychological dimension of procreation precedes and transcends the biology of procreation. Motherhood can be a product of both mental and physical conception; reductionist modes of legal reasoning have ignored this fullness. For the initiating parents, insofar as biology has obfuscated psychology, parental rights have been damaged by misperceptions of parenthood" (Andrea E. Stumpf, "Redefining Mother: A Legal Matrix for New Reproductive Technologies", *The Yale Law Journal* 96 [1986]: 194).

In a somewhat similar vein, Norvin Richards suggests that the commissioner is the person who "takes the actions that start matters biologically" and thus "has parenthood underway": this is "her project", whether she is using a surrogate or an egg donor (Norvin Richards, *The Ethics of Parenthood* [Oxford and New York: Oxford University Press, 2010], 36). Yet if an egg donor, say, advertises her services and then provides her eggs, does she not 'start matters biologically' as much as the commissioning couple, whether or not she *sees* herself as 'having parenthood underway'? And of course, natural parents often find that they are parents without this being a 'project' they have deliberately initiated.

14   Alex Rajczi joins other writers in considering the possibility that biological parents acquire their responsibilities simply by bringing it about that the child is in mortal need. However, he rightly observes that many people:

"feel that the duties of parenthood do not flow from the state of mortal need that the child is in. Instead they flow from the fact that parenthood is a role which carries certain duties with it. In that way it is similar to the role of police officer or citizen, both of which are accompanied by duties beyond the norm" (Rajczi, "Abortion, Competing Entitlements, and Parental Responsibility", 386).

Rajczi comments: "This thought is intuitive, but the problem is that it cannot be expanded into a coherent theory". Recourse to the example of other family roles might have made the task easier: it is puzzling that Rajczi does not address these roles.

15   As Celia Wolf-Devine and Philip E. Devine rightly note:

"the family functions as a bulwark against the instrumentalization of human beings that occurs in the workplace; family members are valued for who they are and not for what they can do. Familial bonds are unchosen, and for that reason provide a safety net for the vulnerable" (Wolf-Devine and Devine, "A Communitarian Pro-Life Perspective", 75).

16   An older sibling may, of course, have 'lobbied' the parents for a new baby, but often this will not be the case. Certainly, the baby will not have lobbied for its own conception and subsequent roles (as child, sibling, grandchild, niece or nephew, etc.).

17   Wreen, "Abortion and Pregnancy Due to Rape", 209.

18   See the comments of "Sarah-Jane":

"It feels like the most natural thing in the world when I see them. I haven't got a maternal bone in my body when it comes to Georgina.

When she cried and I was holding her, I just called for Andrea. Georgina is nothing to do with me, it was my egg and womb, that is all . . . Addiction is usually to drugs or drink but I'm addicted to something healthy—creating families. I certainly don't do this to get rich. I only get money for expenses like maternity clothes, travel costs, extra food. It's the sheer euphoria every time I see the couple so excited that I'm pregnant with their baby. It puts you on a natural high" (Sharon Feinstein, "Celibate Woman Plans to Have 3 Babies", *Mirror*, July 10, 2005, http://www.people.co.uk/archive/other/2005/07/10/celibate-woman-plans-to-have-3-babies-102039–15719946/).

For a less glowing account, see this:

"I had no future; nothing to aspire to or look forward to. My life was mundane and pretty lonely. I thought about surrogacy and the sense of achievement and purpose it would bring. I also considered the bond I would form with the mother; the woman for whom I would carry the baby. She rather than the baby growing inside me, would become the focus of my attention. She would fuss over me and be protective. I would feel valued and valuable . . . I will not have any more children of my own. I do not think I could bond with a baby of my own now. Having deadened my feelings for so long, I do not know if I could feel anything now. I love my own children. I could never, ever part with them. But I do not know what would happen if I tried to have another to keep, for myself. Would I blot out my emotions? Would I be able to distinguish my own child in my womb from a stranger's? I really do not know anymore" (Frances Hardy, "Sarah Fletcher has a vocation: she makes babies for other women", *Daily Mail*, March 23, 1996: 10, http://www.highbeam. com/doc/1G1–111418642.html).

19   Melinda Tankard Reist, "The birth mother not the gestational carrier gave Nic and Keith a baby," http://melindatankardreist.com/2011/01/the-birth-mother-not-the-gestational-carrier-gave-nic-and-keith-a-baby/. Stephen Long points out that: "Just as the womb is not a spaceship, or a submarine, so too we may with a certain wryness observe that it is *not a hospitality suite*, like an extra bedroom in which friends may stay" (Stephen A. Long, *The Teleological Grammar of the Moral Act* [Ave Maria, Florida: Sapientia Press, 2007], 135).

20   Barbara Katz Rothman's comments are of interest here: "Valuing the seed of women, the genetic material women too have, extends to women some of the privileges of patriarchy. That is, when the significance of women's seed is acknowledged in her relationship with her children, women, too, have paternity rights in their children . . . Unlike what happens in a mother-based system, however, this relationship between women and their children is not based on motherhood per se, not on the unique nurturance, the long months of pregnancy, the intimate connections with the baby as it grows and moves inside her body, passes through her genitals, and sucks at her breasts. Instead, women are said to own their babies, have "rights" to them, just as men do: based on their seed . . . Children are, based on the seed, presumptively "half his, half hers"— and might as well have grown in the backyard. Women do not gain their rights to their children in this society as *mothers*, but as *father equivalents*, as equivalent sources of seed" (Rothman, *Recreating Motherhood*, 36–37). Rothman goes on to say that "Upper-class women can have some of the privileges of patriarchy. Upper-class women can have, can buy, some of the privileges of their paternity, using the bodies of poorer women to "bear them offspring" . . . This is the ultimate meaning of patriarch for mothers: seeds are precious; mothers are fungible" (45).

Rothman's points are well taken—though she herself appears to fall into the opposite error of treating motherhood as *entirely* a matter of gestation. Genetic mothers are surely also mothers, even if the new, 'surrogate' mother has taken over the role of 'active mother' and has a right to keep the baby if she wishes.

21   While some surrogates form a close relationship with the commissioning couple, others do not, particularly when the surrogate lives abroad, as can be seen in the following, rather brutal comments of one commissioning mother:

" 'Our baby has no biological connection to the surrogate,' says Octavia.

'Her womb is just the receptacle in which it is being carried. Perhaps it sounds cold and rather clinical, but this is a business transaction. . . .

'Her function is to sustain the foetus we have created. Her blood is pumping around its body and she is feeding it through her placenta, but she is just a vessel. The baby she gives birth to on our behalf will carry none of her genes and bear no physical resemblance to her.

'He or she will have white skin and, in all probability, red hair like my husband.

'Of course I want her to do her best to have a successful pregnancy, and I'll be very upset—quite devastated, in fact—if it doesn't go full-term. But we do not want to get emotionally involved with our surrogate's story. I'm not interested in her background. I don't want to be part of her life.

'She speaks a different language. She lives in a world culturally, economically and socially so remote from ours that the distance between us is unbridgeable. . . .

'I'm assuming that once the baby has popped out and been bathed, he or she will be handed to us. I'm sure the surrogate will see the baby, but she won't breastfeed it or cuddle it.

'We may briefly see our surrogate, too, and I will thank her. I'm certain she will have formed a bond with the baby—no woman who has carried a baby for nine months could fail to do so—but I do not anticipate there will be any problems handing it over. I've no worries. She certainly won't want to extend her own family.' "

Helen Roberts and Frances Hardy, "Our 'rent a womb' child from an Indian baby farm", *Daily Mail*, August 31, 2012 (updated September 1, 2012), http://www.dailymail.co.uk/femail/article-2196538/Our-rent-womb-child-Indian-baby-farm-British-couple-paying-20–000-desperately-poor-single-mother-child.html#ixzz26AEYdVBN.

22 Cecile Fabre describes situations where the surrogate may come to care for the child's welfare and relinquish him or her to the commissioning couple not simply for the money, but because she sees the couple as better able to care for the child than she is herself (Cecile Fabre, *Whose Body Is It Anyway?* [Oxford: Clarendon, 2006], 210–11). While this could certainly happen, there is little recognition shown by Fabre of the sadness and distortion it involves: a woman effectively assumes what is arguably a maternal role (whether or not she sees it as such when she assumes it), which she then feels ill-equipped to carry through on by deciding to keep the baby. Relevant here may be a fact to which Fabre herself explicitly draws attention: some surrogates have low self-esteem, and may take on surrogate motherhood as a way of atoning for what they see as mistaken decisions in the past, such as abortion or even adoption (Fabre, *Whose Body*, 192, 199–200, 203).

23 See, e.g., Rosalyn Diprose, *The Bodies of Women* (London: Routledge, 1994), 117: "To hold a surrogate to her contract is to assume that the product of her labour is not part of herself". Note the use of the word "part" to refer even to the newborn baby.

24 Fabre rightly points out that those who transfer responsibility for a child will be transferring only those rights they *have* over the child, which are not rights of ownership (Fabre, *Whose Body is it Anyway?* 190). She argues that surrogates do not regard children as commodities (mostly), whereas, in her view, celebrity couples who sold their one-year-olds for substantial sums would so regard them (Fabre, 191). It is not clear how Fabre is able to make such a sharp distinction here. In any event, Fabre appears to accept that children are bought and sold in surrogacy: she says frankly that "the fact that surrogacy may indeed involve the sale and purchase of babies does not suffice to render it impermissible" (Fabre, 213).

25 See the following chapter for some examples.

26 Gheaus, "The Right to Parent One's Biological Baby". This position is very widely accepted, including by such authors as Gregory Kaebnick—who otherwise suggests in somewhat dualistic vein that genetic testing "establishes one, narrow, biological *kind* of parenthood—not a relationship between persons,

but one between organisms" (Gregory E. Kaebnick, "The Natural Father: Genetic Paternity Testing, Marriage, and Fatherhood", *Cambridge Quarterly of Healthcare Ethics* 13 [2004], 55).

27 See Anca Gheaus: "There are two general features of real-world pregnancies that speak in favour of adequate parents' moral right to keep their birth babies. First, pregnancies involve a variety of costs—physical, psychological, social and financial. Most of these costs can only be shouldered by pregnant women and, to some extent, their supportive partner. Second, during pregnancy many—perhaps most—expectant parents form a poignantly embodied, but also emotional, intimate relationship with their fetus. The two features are related, because this relationship is fostered by bearing parents' willingness to take on the costs of pregnancy and by their actual experience of its burdens. These two features of pregnancy can, given a fundamental right to parent in general, ground a parent-interest based right to keep one's birth baby" (Gheaus, "The Right to Parent One's Biological Baby", 15).

28 Gerald H. Paske, "Sperm-napping and the Right Not to Have a Child," *Australasian Journal of Philosophy* 6.1 (1987): 98–103.

29 Note that genetic motherhood, like genetic fatherhood, has a certain pattern which is not reproduced in cloning, where the genetic link is much closer. Genetic mothers do not, like clone originals, provide almost all the offspring's genetic input, but merely some of that input—in collaboration with genetic fathers and in a way randomized pre-fertilization during the process of 'meiosis'. This combination of genetic novelty and genetic familiarity surely has value for both child and parents: the child is both anchored in the past and launched towards a future which is very much his or her own.

30 Cecile Fabre, who supports surrogacy, nonetheless opposes surrogacy contracts seeking to prevent the pregnant woman from bonding with, i.e., loving, the baby she is carrying (Fabre, *Whose Body Is It Anyway?* 198–9).

31 "Connie Sellars", in *Victims and Victors: Speaking Out About Their Pregnancies, Abortions, and Children Resulting from Sexual Assault,* eds. David C. Reardon, Julie Makimaa, Amy Sobie (Springfield, IL: Acorn Books, 2000), 91–2. For a comprehensive indictment of social attitudes to rape victims who become pregnant and choose to keep the child, see Shauna R. Prewitt, "Giving Birth to a "Rapist's Child": A Discussion and Analysis of the Limited Legal Protections Afforded to Women Who Become Mothers Through Rape," *Georgetown Law Journal* 98 (2010): 827–62. In fact, almost a third of U.S. women who conceive via rape choose to keep the child, rather than abort it or give it up for adoption (M.M. Holmes, H.S. Resnick, D.G. Kilpatrick, and C.L. Best, "Rape-related Pregnancy: Estimates and Descriptive Characteristics from a National Sample of Women", *American Journal of Obstetrics and Gynecology* 175.2 (1996): 320–4; discussion 324–5). A study carried out by Rape Crisis Network Ireland of rape victims who became pregnant found that a majority not only gave birth to, but chose to keep their babies (Rape Crisis Network, Ireland, "What does RCNI National Data Collection tell us about rape survivors and termination of pregnancy?" http://www.rcni.ie/uploads/RangeOfOutcomesOfSurvivorsOfRapeWhoArePregnantAsAResultOfRape2011.pdf).

32 Compare Hilde Lindemann Nelson: "Pregnancy is not just something that attaches to women; it is not like a coat or a haircut. On the contrary, once she becomes aware of the pregnancy, a woman often takes it to be a centrally important fact about herself. If the pregnancy is an unwanted intrusion—the product of rape, for example—the woman might experience it as an external fact that has nothing to do with who she is. But a feature can be both central

and something one distances oneself from, as for example a person might repudiate his ethnic heritage and embrace that of the dominant culture. The raped pregnant woman will probably try to put the pregnancy outside her internal point of view, but I do not think she will altogether succeed unless she terminates the pregnancy. In that sense her pregnancy is a part of her inner perspective, motivating her to reorient herself and to take action in a way that it cannot do for those looking on from the outside" (Nelson, "The Architect and the Bee", 264).

This account neglects to note the possibility—and actuality for many women—of responding to a role that already exists and has its own, objective moral demands. By analogy, a woman who realizes that she is lactating and that her newborn needs her to breastfeed is not *creating* the significance of lactation and breastfeeding *ex nihilo* but *recognizing and personalizing* this significance in her nurturing response. So too with pregnancy: the woman 'creates' her actual response at the psychological level, but does not 'create' the moral demand for a nurturing, non-destructive response to her baby's needs.

33 "Connie Sellars", in *Victims and Victors*, 91.
34 Ibid., 92.
35 Mary Murray, in *Victims and Victors*, 81.
36 Sharon "Bailey", in *Victims and Victors*, 86.
37 Ibid., 89.
38 Kathleen DeZeeuw, in *Victims and Victors*, 76: "I was really pregnant! Words can never truly describe the horror this brought me.
    However, once the baby continued to kick and move, I began to have different feelings towards the child. I began to realise that this little life inside me was struggling too. Somehow, my heart changed. I was no longer thinking of the baby as the "rapist's". Maternal bonding began in this 16-year-old girl. To this day that, too, is hard to describe.
    I no longer wanted to abort this child . . . When I was sent to the home in Michigan, an even stronger bond developed between me and the child. I now thought of the baby as "my baby". My baby was all that I had. I felt abandoned by everyone. I had only the life inside me to talk to. It was just us two."
39 Kathleen DeZeeuw, in *Victims and Victors*, 74–80.
40 Ibid., 79.
41 Mary Rosera Joyce's words are of interest here, in describing the possibility of actively and positively acknowledging an initially unwanted pregnancy as a change to one's 'being' (or at least, we might say, as the start of a radically new mental-physical state and role):
    "A woman begins to control her own mind when she moves from doing to being, and asks herself, 'Who am I in this situation?' She knows she is pregnant and doesn't want to be. She knows that pregnancy makes her a mother. If she denies that she is already a mother, she makes a statement about her pregnancy and herself. If she thinks she is pregnant with a piece of growing tissue similar to a tumor, she belittles pregnancy and diminishes herself, as the playboy mentality would have her do. But if she thinks she is pregnant with another being of her own kind, her person and her sexuality immediately have more dignity in her own eyes. She might say, 'I suppose I *am* a mother whether or not I want to be. Just as I am myself whether or not I want to be . . . What kind of mother am I going to be: one who receives my motherhood and gives birth to my child, or one who denies it and removes what I am carrying?'. . .
    As a woman gains control of her mind in this way, she does not passively, helplessly, let her situation tell her whether or not she is a mother. She does not let her wanting or unwanting tell her who she is. She lets her being inform her

mind and her decision. She decides to become *receptive* instead of remaining a passive victim of circumstances. 'I choose to receive my being as a mother. I choose to receive my situation and make the best of it somehow. My situation is not going to tell me that I should not be who I am'. When she receives her situation, it becomes a challenge to her being, no longer just an imposition. She can now respond to the challenge according to the kind of person she *really prefers* to be" (Joyce, "Are Women Controlling Their Own Minds?" 233–4).

Note that 'associating' oneself willingly with a pregnancy need not (as some assume) presuppose access to abortion; on the contrary, some such willing association even with very demanding pregnancies seems if anything more common in societies *without* the ready access to abortion which in Western-ized societies has done so much to build resentment and alienate women from their babies.

42 The suffering caused to the mother by adopting out a child is sometimes used to argue for abortion or even, more recently, infanticide (see note 4 of Chapter 2).

43 "Because in giving a child up for adoption one ceases to be the child's carer but does not cease to be the child's progenitor; and because causing a child to exist generates obligations towards that child; birth parents are, in an impor-tant sense, always parents come what may" (Lindsey Porter, "Adoption Is Not Abortion-Lite", *Journal of Applied Philosophy* 29.1 [2012]: 63). Porter rightly argues that there are cases—such as when the adoptive family becomes destitute—when it simply will not do to say "I'm not the parent anymore" (72).

44 It is true that an existing commitment and pattern of sexual behavior will sometimes involve some form of general consent to parenthood, whether or not a particular sexual act had that intention. Whether couples might prepare better for pregnancy, in relation to both means and circumstances of (planned or possible) conception, is a question we will explore in the next chapter.

45 Celia Wolf-Devine and Philip E. Devine point out that "Not only does eas-ily available abortion encourage men to feel disconnected from and not responsible for their own offspring, but it also lets the broader society off the hook for stepping in and doing what is necessary for poor children. And the individualistic philosophy promoted by pro-choice people, which denies our responsibility to care for even the children we ourselves brought into being, undercuts every possible response to the complaints of taxpayers about being made to pay for other people's irresponsibly begotten children" (Wolf-Devine and Devine, "A Communitarian Pro-Life Perspective", 98).

Fritz Oehlschlaeger similarly notes the privatization of childbearing and childrearing as a consequence of treating pregnancy as supererogatory (despite the fact that most women do in practice carry their babies to term). Oehlsch-laeger suggests that as childbearing ceases to be the norm,

"it becomes necessary rhetorically to present children as resources in order to make claims on public funding necessary for education and social welfare. Self-interested maximizers who see childbearing as extraordinary will quite appropriately expect their support for other people's children to yield a return. It seems inevitable that children will come to seem private commodities at home—where they must satisfy parents convinced of their own heroism in even venturing to have children—and resources available for others' use in their public lives" (Fritz Oehlschlaeger, *Procreative Ethics: Philosophical and Christian Approaches to Questions at the Beginning of Life* [Eugene, OR: Cascade Books, 2010], 146–7).

46   See, for example, Elizabeth Brake, "Fatherhood and Child Support: Do Men Have a Right to Choose?" *Journal of Applied Philosophy* 22.1 (2005): 55–70. Contrast Mary Catherine Sommers:

"Parenting . . . is a task towards which the resources of a whole society should be turned. But one cannot argue consistently both that the decision to extend bodily life support to one's offspring is simply the discretionary use of one's body for a personal project and, that others, from the father of the child to one's fellow-citizens, are bound to support this project in various capacities. One could argue that in a society which, consistent with its individualistic principles, has de facto shifted ultimate responsibility for offspring to those who physically bear them, there is no other way to return to a communal sense of responsibility unless women abandon or refuse the burden. The short answer to this is that revolution, like war, has its rules: it should not be waged on the innocent. . . ." (Sommers, "Living Together", 251).

In similar vein, Celia Wolf-Devine and Philip E. Devine observe that "Women are not, by virtue of their oppression, entitled to pursue their interests without regard to the interests and rights of others. If feminism is merely a movement to pursue the interests of women at all costs, it loses the moral high ground and becomes one lobby among many" (Wolf-Devine and Devine, "A Communitarian Pro-Life Perspective", 95).

47   Elizabeth Brake points out that child support payments "might make it difficult for [a man] to **start a family** [emphasis added] or pursue other important plans", and that as "some occupations involve physical risk, the burdens of mandatory child support and of pregnancy might sometimes be comparable. It seems difficult to justify a general claim that the burdens of pregnancy are always greater than those of working overtime for eighteen years in a risky environment—or, for a chronically unemployed man under a system of stringent enforcement, those of destitution, possible imprisonment, and mounting arrears" (Brake, "Fatherhood and Child Support", 65).

48   See Elizabeth Brake: "Pregnancy, like disease transmission, is a proximate effect of sex; childbirth is determined by further steps, the woman's choice" (63). It is striking that Brake compares pregnancy successively to (a) disease transmission, and (b) being mauled by bears while walking through a bear park—despite having first applied bear spray (62–63). Such comparisons are telling in that they omit not only the value of the new life conceived but the goal-directed nature of intercourse for the couple: intercourse is biologically *aimed* at conception in a way that walking about is not aimed at being mauled by bears (even if bears may aim at mauling!).

49   Even a rapist may rightly be regarded as a father, though normally a father with particular narrow duties (i.e., to pay child support) but no obvious rights or *social* duties vis-à-vis the child. Having said that, a rapist father might have some responsibility to agree to some form of contact should the child (in particular, an older child) desire this, and should the mother permit it. One case of such contact is recorded in *Victims and Victors* (88), though the girl's mother has very natural reservations, despite the man's contrition for the rape. On the trauma and injustice involved in legally forcing the raped woman to allow the rapist access to the child she is raising, see Shauna R. Prewitt, "Giving Birth to a 'Rapist's Child'."

50   In her paper "Pleading Men and Virtuous Women: Considering the Role of the Father in the Abortion Debate" (*International Journal of Applied Philosophy* 21.1 [2007]: 15), Bertha Manninen suggests that "A woman who brings a fetus, whom she initially wanted to abort, to term in order to give a good man a chance to be a good father is courageous, fair, kind, empathetic, selfless,

and **very noble indeed**" (emphasis added). While many will agree that this is a virtuous choice, some will add that it is a minimally decent choice (the two not being incompatible). On the next page, Manninen comments that "Perhaps after much deliberation and consideration of the man's position, a woman may still decide that she cannot face the prospect of **adopting out** her child [emphasis added], even if it is to the infant's father. Perhaps she knows that if she does continue to gestate, she too would become engrossed in the fetus and in the future child, and this is *precisely* what she does not want."

Manninen's concern for the suffering of men in this situation is welcome. However, in taking what appears still an 'ownership' approach to the mother-fetus relationship, she underestimates the duties of the pregnant woman to a worrying degree. The man's situation can perhaps be compared to that of a woman separated from her newborn—let's say, because she is incarcerated—who pleads with the father not to kill the baby to avoid social fatherhood but rather to care for it until she gets out and can do so herself. The oddity of Manninen's description of the father of the unborn child being 'invited in' to 'adopt' his own baby should also be noted: the man does not need to *assume* parental rights and duties which already exist—though how these might be integrated with the woman's own parental rights and duties would need to be carefully hammered out.

In situations in which the woman legally, if not emotionally, holds all the cards in relation to the unborn child's survival, men's emotional abdication is both encouraged by and encourages the woman's own retreat from parenthood. Personal testimonies of post-abortion grief from men, as well as women, can be found readily on-line; see, e.g., Phil McCombs, "Remembering Thomas" *The American Feminist* 5.1 (1998): 11, at http://www.feministsfor life.org/remembering-thomas/.

51 Of interest here is the following reflection from an anti-abortion campaigner: "Traditionally, manhood was defined by a number of things. Men were supposed to be loyal, courageous, responsible, and above all, willing to sacrifice for those they had a duty to protect—namely, women and children. This protective instinct was considered to be as natural as the female maternal instinct . . . Today, popular culture seems to measure manhood up against how many women a man has slept with.

When debating others, I have often found myself facing this same "ideal." One university student asked how I was a man if I wasn't sleeping with "chicks," to which I informed him that I held to the quaint point of view that it took more of a man to keep one woman happy for a lifetime than dozens for ten minutes.

When I was doing "Choice" Chain on the streets of Vancouver with two of my pro-life friends, one middle-aged man walked past and asked us, "Shouldn't you guys be out trying to get laid or something?" This actually shocked me. Whether or not you agree with our position, surely it is more admirable to defend your beliefs in your free time rather than trying to "get laid."

This is why catch phrases such as "pro-choice" are heralded by many men with such ferocity. "Pro-choice" to them doesn't just mean the woman's right to kill her pre-born child; it also means "pro-choice" regarding whether or not men have to stick around and care for the offspring they fathered.

One of my friends who regularly pickets abortion clinics has informed me that we would be shocked to see how many sobbing girls are pushed into abortion clinics by their angry boyfriends and fathers. When picketing in front of the Edmonton abortion clinic, I noticed boyfriends driving up, dropping their girlfriends off, and then promptly leaving. Perhaps more women would stop being "pro-choice" about killing pre-born children if the fathers of these children would stop being "pro-choice" about actually shouldering their responsibilities, as has been the tradition of true manhood in the past.

That some men think that sex is purely recreational and has no consequences is imbecilic and delusional." Jonathon Van Maren, "Men and Abortion: The Forgotten Accomplices", http://www.unmaskingchoice.ca/blog/2011/09/23/men-and-abortion-forgotten-accomplices.

52 In the words of Hilda Lindeman Nelson, "The pregnant woman is . . . doing something in the present moment for the fetus she carries. Here the simile with the architect is particularly apt, for what she is doing is using her body to make a home. This too is an activity that involves far more than blind uncomprehending nature. A tree in a rainstorm can be said to offer shelter only in a metaphorical sense, but a woman does it quite literally with her body. She extends bodily hospitality first, in intercourse, to the man who fathers the child, then to the growing fetus, then later perhaps to the baby who suckles at her breast" (Nelson, "The Architect and the Bee", 264).

Nelson is right to say that "Human pregnancy is no more purely biological than any other human activity" (Nelson, "The Architect and the Bee", 262). Yet Nelson underestimates the significance of the 'given', pre-conscious side of pregnancy: any pregnancy, like any human life, involves many bodily activities of which the woman is unaware throughout the pregnancy—not just while she is asleep, and before she knows of the pregnancy, but throughout its entire course. More importantly, the shelter and nurture pregnancy provides has a biological-social meaning waiting to be discovered: the woman does not need to 'inject' meaning into a 'purely biological' process that somehow lacks all meaning of its own.

53 Cecilia Cancellaro, *Pregnancy Stories: Real Women Share the Joys, Fears, Thrills, and Anxieties of Pregnancy from Conception to Birth* (Oakland, CA: New Harbinger, 2001), 27, cit Mullin, *Reconceiving*, 29.

54 Mullin, *Reconceiving*, 66.

55 Schueneman, "Creating Life, Giving Birth, and Learning to Die", 169. Schueneman refers earlier to "the paradoxical feeling of gaining power while losing control" (168).

56 See, for example, these recommendations on the parenting website parentingweekly.com, in an article entitled "Making the Best of Bed Rest":

"You may find yourself feeling jealous of your friends or partner for being able to lead normal, active lives while you are shut in. You may also feel intense loneliness, isolation, helplessness, boredom, guilt, and fear. These feelings are all normal and be prepared to have some bad days. Don't hesitate to reach out to your close friends, family, partner, and religious or professional counselors if you are feeling desperate. Try to stay positive and focused on the goal: delivering a healthy baby. Keep in mind that every day she is still inside you is a victory, and the better her chances for survival. Hang an ultrasound picture of your baby where you can see it and use it as a focal point for meditation and a constant reminder of why you are doing all this. Take advantage of this time to bond with your unborn baby. You will probably be able to feel every poke, turn, and hiccup more acutely than other mothers-to-be who may be on the run and too busy to notice. Try to think of this time as a special opportunity to sing, talk, and read to your baby" (http://www.parentingweekly.com/pregnancy/pregnancy-complications/making-the-best-of-bedrest_2.htm).

57 Julie Piering, "The Pregnant Body as a Public Body: An Occasion for Community Care, Instrumental Coercion, and a Singular Collectivity", in *Philosophical Inquiries into Pregnancy, Childbirth, and Mothering*, eds. Sheila Lintott and Maureen Sander-Staudt (New York: Routledge, 2012), 179.

58 Piering, "The Pregnant Body", 186–7.

59 Regarding the 'watchfulness' society requires in relation to pregnant women, Piering comments that:

"This watchfulness might be a friend, family member, or kindly waiter who informs a pregnant woman of research on the perils of alfalfa sprouts in time to prevent her from ordering a certain sandwich. Rather than undermining her subjectivity by treating her as a problematic body, this considerate attention seeks to provide her with important information and support the project, pregnancy, in which she is engaged. . . . Mean-spirited finger wagging and demeaning disapproval by poorly behaved strangers may have the best interest of the child in mind, but it is hard to imagine that it achieves its goal . . . Given the injustice done to Carrie Buck and other victims of compulsory sterilization policies in the U.S., we would do well to think through the real grounds of social evaluations regarding the fitness of potential mothers. While mindful of this, there is a care and watchfulness that can be afforded a pregnant woman that supports her subjectivity, is given in a spirit of generosity and creates an atmosphere of mutuality. This, I take it, benefits the pregnant woman, her future child, and the community at large" (Piering, "The Pregnant Body as a Public Body", 184–5).

60 Smajdor, "The Moral Imperative for Ectogenesis", 340–1.

61 Stephen D. Schwartz, *The Moral Question of Abortion* (Chicago: Loyola University Press, 1990), 212, cit. Beckwith, *Defending Life*, 170.

62 Parental neglect of a child after birth will also—though in different ways— involve a failure to use one's body to care properly for the child.

63 Note the difference here: even if a cesarian section is needed to protect the woman's health as well as the baby's, it is widely agreed that we should not inflict one on a competent woman without her consent (for contrary views, see Carol Tauer, "Lives at Stake: How to Respond to a Woman's Refusal of Cesarian Surgery When She Risks Losing Her Child or Her Life", *Health Progress* [Sept 1992]: 20–27; Julian Savulescu, "Future People, Involuntary Medical Treatment in Pregnancy and the Duty of Easy Rescue", *Utilitas* 19 [2007]: 1–20). In contrast, as Savulescu notes, we do sometimes impose treatment in other contexts to avert risks to third parties; for example, treatment of an unwilling, competent mentally ill person who is a danger to others, or of a competent person unwilling to be treated for an infectious disease. The difference with cesarians is striking, and can be linked to the special role that pregnancy constitutes: the woman is 'custodian' or 'guardian' of her unborn child in a way the mental patient or infectious patient is not custodian of those who might be affected.

64 This theme was famously explored by Barbara Katz Rothman in *The Tentative Pregnancy* (New York: Penguin, 1986).

65 Such adjustment may extend to the couple's sexual choices: couples at high risk of miscarriage, for example, should consider abstaining from intercourse while the woman is pregnant. Similarly, those spacing children with hormonal contraception, which can endanger early embryos, should pursue other, non-abortifacient means. 'Natural family planning', in particular, is safe and effective in standard modern versions, though it does involve abstinence on fertile days of the woman's menstrual cycle.

66 Mullin, *Reconceiving*, 73. See also Rothman, *Recreating Motherhood*, 21: "One New York City subway ad series shows two newborn footprints, one from a full-term and one from a premature infant. The ads read, 'Guess which baby's mother smoked while pregnant?' Another asks, 'Guess which baby's mother drank while pregnant?' And yet another: 'Guess which baby's mother

didn't get prenatal care?' I look in vain for the ad that says 'Guess which baby's mother tried to get by on welfare?'; 'Guess which baby's mother had to live on the streets?'; or 'Guess which baby's mother was beaten by her husband?'"

67   Melinda Tankard Reist, Defiant Birth: Women Who Resist Medical Eugenics (Melbourne: Spinifex Press, 2006). See also Rothman, *The Tentative Pregnancy*.

68   For example, the woman may be offered footprints or photographs of her baby, as in the case of natural stillbirth. While the fetus is not seen as a baby for the purpose of respecting the life abortion targets, paradoxically it *is* seen as a baby for the purpose of mourning the child when it is dead.

69   The interest in continuing to live is, of course, only one human interest; other 'human goods' such as friendship, knowledge and play can also normally be promoted in disabled children, not least by promoting life itself, the prerequisite for all of them.

70   Note that even those who accept (non-voluntary) euthanasia of born disabled children may be less willing to accept it for some conditions for which abortion is routinely offered (Down Syndrome, spina bifida, hemophilia).

71   Health professionals may feel under pressure to free State resources by enabling abortion, or may simply be unwilling to acknowledge that children with certain conditions have lives of genuine value to themselves and their families, even though the condition may not be amenable to treatment.

72   The claim here is that once a child is conceived, to be unable to bring that child successfully to term is not only a failure in the pregnant woman's healthy functioning—already a disvalue—but a failure in health or 'functionality', at least while the child remains within her. This is so whatever the cause of the woman's inability: the fact she has just taken an abortion drug, for example, may mean that she is now unable (at least without medical reversal) to bring her still-living child to term, although previously she was able. Of course, a woman's health, including her reproductive health, could be excellent without her actually conceiving in the first place (say, because she is celibate, or her partner is infertile). I explore these issues further in "Life and Health: A Value in Itself for Human Beings?"

73   Susan Mattingly neglects the possibility of such a reproductive health interest, and sees a legitimate focus on the woman's "protective biological and social role" as "looking beyond the maternal patient" (Susan S. Mattingly, "The Maternal-Fetal Dyad: Exploring the Two-Patient Obstetric Model", *Hastings Center Report* [January–February 1992]: 17). While Mattingly is right to draw attention to the moral relevance of any social burdens of the treatment itself for the woman and her family (for example, lack of funds for that treatment), less benign is her suggestion that the very survival of a new family member could be reasonably seen as a 'social' bad: "increasing the chances for live delivery of a severely damaged fetus . . . might be a medical value but a family disvalue" (18–19). We should not see a disabled family member in these terms: the presence of the disabled child (or older person) can put pressure on the family —not least when the family is not well supported —but in itself, that presence is a family value, not a family disvalue. This is so even if the disabled child's care is endangering the health of the parents or other family members: it would be unconscionable to treat this as a reason to engineer the disabled child's death, rather than offer that child and the family more support.

74   When speaking of risks and harms we need to factor in the woman's reproductive health interest in giving birth to a live baby and retaining her fertility—so if we are comparing, say, a cesarian to a live organ donation, we would need

to imagine an organ donation which somehow also had the effect of promoting the health of any child the donor subsequently conceived. Such benefits would not, however, justify organ donation, or a cesarian, where the risk and/or harm to the immediate subject was simply too high.

A question arises whether, just as the woman has a biological interest in giving birth to a live baby, a baby has a biological interest in being born without ending the life of its (presumptive) primary carer. Certainly, the baby has a substantial social interest in its mother's survival; however, whether it has a *biological* interest in this survival is more moot. The situations are not symmetric, as the fetus is internal to the woman and caught up in her reproductive health, in a way the woman is not internal to, but rather the 'person-environment of', her unborn child. Having said that, a baby with an outsized head which will make vaginal birth very difficult is at least arguably disabled, just like a baby born without the ability to breastfeed. Mother and baby are perhaps best seen as having a joint biological-and-social interest in a safe pregnancy and birth, although their overall health interests can diverge in high-risk situations. (Note that such divergence can have moral implications of a kind that do not touch on abortion: positive interventions to maintain a pregnancy—let's say, an ectopic pregnancy—will be counterindicated if we are more likely to harm the woman than to promote her health by enabling the pregnancy to continue. Here as elsewhere, any actual interventions on the woman herself would need to be in her interests overall—or, at least, not very harmful to her.)

75 The woman might even regret having had IVF, but nonetheless feel responsible for her remaining embryos and believe that in helping her begin their nurture her doctor would be doing something medically appropriate. See the next chapter for a discussion of IVF and the predicament of frozen embryos.

76 Garcia, "Intentions in Medical Ethics"; J.L.A. Garcia, "The Doubling Undone? Double Effect in Recent Medical Ethics", *Philosophical Papers* 36.2 (2007): 245–70.

77 "Two-patient benefit-burden transactions require of physicians a deferential approach to those asked to assume medical risks for others and a readiness to shield reluctant or indecisive patients from involuntary harm. If the example of transplantation ethics is followed in obstetrics, physicians have acquired obligations to neutralize moral pressures on pregnant women arising from family relationships and ensure that any maternal sacrifices to benefit the fetus are strictly voluntary" (Mattingly, "The Maternal-Fetal Dyad", 16–17).

78 See the website www.cancerinpregnancy.org.

79 Any waiving by the woman of her rights in this area should be seen as just that: a waiving of a right to treatment to which she is morally entitled. It should also be distinguished from any authorization of lethal invasions of the woman's own body—invasions of a kind one is arguably not entitled to authorize, even to save a family member (see below).

80 On conjoined twin separation dilemmas, see Watt, "Conjoined Twins". Again, the case of conjoined twins can be helpful in thinking through prenatal conflicts between twins more generally: twins who are not (otherwise) conjoined can share a placenta during pregnancy to which they are linked by separate umbilical cords, and this can create the serious medical condition of fetus-to-fetus blood transfusion, where the exchange of blood between twins is not equal (one twin sends more to the placenta than it gets back, and vice versa).

One medical response of attempting to isolate the area of placenta each twin uses, even if risky, may be ethically acceptable, as offering the best hope of bringing both to term. In contrast, a much more problematic response is to block the umbilical cord of one twin so that it cannot function, and thus cannot affect the blood supply of the other—though the twin whose cord is blocked will die. This would be a deliberate (and lethal) bodily invasion of the twin who is targeted to benefit his or her sibling—rather like cutting the windpipe of someone whose breathing is endangering another person. As such, it would, I believe, be morally excluded, even if death of the first twin as such (as opposed to dysfunction of his or her body-part, the umbilical cord) is not intended.

81 These issues are the subject of intense debate, in which two quite different questions are often not addressed separately: whether death (or harm or dysfunction) need be intended when carrying out a bodily invasion one knows will result in death; and whether, despite the possible absence of any such intention, the intended bodily invasion takes place in 'circumstances'—if that is the correct term—which are conclusive for the moral categorization of the act.

Works that address the categorisation of bodily invasions such as 'craniotomy' (a procedure where the baby's skull is crushed, still used in some countries in cases of obstructed labor) include John Finnis, Germain Grisez and Joseph Boyle, "'Direct' and 'Indirect': A Reply to Critics of Our Action Theory", *Thomist* 65.1 (2001): 1–44 (note that these authors explicitly recognize that there are other possible objections to such interventions besides the putative intention to cause death). For a more recent defence of such interventions, see Martin Rhonheimer, *Vital Conflicts in Medical Ethics: A Virtue Approach to Craniotomy and Tubal Pregnancies* (Washington, DC: Catholic University of America Press, 2009). For a different approach, where these kinds of intervention are opposed without imputing a necessary intention to cause death, see, e.g., J. L. A. Garcia, "Intentions in Medical Ethics," in *Human Lives: Critical Essays on Consequentialist Bioethics*, eds. David Oderberg and Jacqueline Laing (London: Macmillan, 1997), 164–66; Stephen Brock, *Action & Conduct: Thomas Aquinas and the Theory of Action* (Edinburgh: T&T Clark, 1998); Anthony McCarthy, "Unintended Morally Determinative Aspects (UMDAs): Moral Absolutes, Moral Acts and Physical Features in Reproductive and Sexual Ethics" (*Studia Philosophiae Christianae* 51.2 (2015), 143–158); Helen Watt, "Beyond Double Effect: Side-effects and Bodily Harm", in *Human Values: New Essays on Ethics and Natural Law*, eds. David Oderberg and Timothy Chappell (London: Palgrave MacMillan, 2004), 236–51.

82 In contrast, simply breathing oneself as best one can while foreseeing that this will mean less oxygen for the other person would be a different kind of choice.

83 I am leaving aside other problematic issues such as arrest and punishment for past offences, as we are here describing private acts of self-defence or defence of another.

84 The term is taken from McCarthy, "Unintended Morally Determinative Aspects (UMDAs)."

85 Note that it is standard in double-effect reasoning to see side-effects as morally relevant in the sense that they must be proportionate to intended gains. Here I am making the separate point that *some* side-effects or unintended aspects of *some* intentions are morally conclusive in combination with those intentions.

86 According to the 'principle of totality,' a traditional principle in medical ethics, we should look to harms and benefits within the good of health when assessing whether an intervention counts as mutilation and should therefore be avoided as harmful to the subject. An amputation, for example, will inevitably cause loss of function as a side-effect but this harm may be greatly outweighed by the benefits for the overall health of the patient.

87 I am referring here to a bodily invasion which is not only harmful, but would harm even a healthy person of the relevant age. In contrast, if an intervention that would be harmless to a healthy person would harm a dying person—let's say, opening his clenched jaws to remove a whistle needed to attract rescuers' attention—this might be permissible in extremis even if the person's death would be foreseeably brought forward (see the discussion at the end of this chapter of post-viability early delivery of babies with lethal anomalies).

88 For example, we could think of a contract killer, whose knowledge that his victim is innocent is hardly a *mere* circumstance, even if the person is not killed precisely qua innocent person, but as someone a customer wants dead. Other examples readily suggest themselves: the victim's lack of consent in rape is not a mere circumstance but definitive of the rapist's act. Even if the rapist does not care if the victim consents or not, he is not doing 'the same thing' as he would in a case of consensual sex but with the added 'circumstance' (in the sense of something external to the act itself) that consent is lacking.

89 I am not referring here to 'peri-mortem cesarians' in which the woman's heart has stopped, and relieving the pressure on her by delivering her viable fetus has the aim of saving her own life, and not just her child's.

90 The 'reproductive health interest' in delivering a live baby would here be subsumed by the general health interest in surviving (and if possible recovering from) birth—bearing in mind that if a woman is seriously injured, even if she is not literally made sterile, this too affects her reproductive health.

91 Note that this scenario is evidence against the claim that the pregnant woman and fetus are really one organism. If that were truly the case, there would be no dilemma here (at least in the case of a woman who was not competent to request or refuse the procedure), since the supposed 'single organism' would benefit from the excising of the 'part' (here, the adult 'part') that could not be saved for the benefit of the supposed whole.

92 See Watt, *Life and Death in Healthcare Ethics,* 32–6.

93 A woman with cancer she has a good chance of treating successfully, though at the cost of the lives of her twin babies, is not, or so most of us believe, morally obliged to forgo cancer treatment, such as a hysterectomy, which she urgently needs. Such cases make it clear that moral decision-making in this area is not simply a question of 'counting lives saved' (which is not to say that additional lives saved need not be factored into the woman's decision e.g. to wait a little longer if she can).

94 Kevin Flannery, "Vital Conflicts and the Catholic Magisterial Tradition," *National Catholic Bioethics Quarterly* 11.4 (2011): 702–4. Flannery regards such a hypothetical intervention as similar to the cutting out of a diseased fallopian tube—or to a mountain-climber cutting off his own leg in a desperate attempt to free himself from a dangling companion to whom he is tightly bound. On the role of the placenta and abortion methods, see Jay J. Bringman and Robert B. Shabanowitz, "The Placenta as an Organ of the Fetus", *National Catholic Bioethics Quarterly* 15 (2015): 31–37. See also subsequent discussion of this paper in the journal; for example, in the following issue 15.2 (2015): Peter J. Cataldo, William Cusick, Becket Gremmels et al., "Deplantation of the Placenta in Maternal-Fetal Vital Conflicts"; John A. DiCamillo and Edward J. Furton, "Early Induction and Double Effect"; Nicanor Austriaco, "Resolving Crisis Pregnancies: Acting on the Mother versus Acting on the Fetal Child". On using the mother's own contractions rather than instruments to extract the fetus in a way that similarly itself endangers its life, see note 23 of Chapter 2.

95 Admittedly, the term is often used in a technical sense and with a qualifier: 'material' aggressor.

96　Ectopic pregnancies may be found in other parts of the body such as the abdomen and in very rare cases can be surgically delivered after viability.

97　Fernandez Hervé, Perrine Capmas et al., "Fertility After Ectopic Pregnancy: The DEMETER Randomized Trial", *Human Reproduction* 28 (2013): 1247–53.

98　The trophoblast is the developmental precursor to the placenta.

99　Note that the embryo will often already have died, even if the trophoblastic tissue may remain and continue to divide. An isolated part of an organism is not an organism, and persisting trophoblastic tissue may be attacked in any way that is most effective.

100　Such damage may be particularly likely with modern laparoscopic or 'keyhole' techniques—a point made by Christopher Kaczor ("The Ethics of Ectopic Pregnancy: A Critical Reconsideration of Salpingostomy and Methotrexate", *Linacre Quarterly* 76.3 [2009]: 265–82). Kaczor suggests that if, with older, more 'open' surgical techniques, it is possible to contemplate transplanting the embryo to the womb, a procedure claimed to have been done by several doctors, this must mean that deliberate removal of the embryo from the tube is not in itself morally proscribed. This is, however, to presume that the 'circumstance' that the embryo is not, in standard practice, being moved to a safer place in its mother's body is a *mere* circumstance, rather than a morally determinative albeit unintended aspect of the action— see the discussion above. (Similarly with MTX, Kaczor appears to treat the fact that a trophoblast might belong to a still-living rather than a now-deceased embryo as a 'mere' circumstance of using MTX to stop damage by the trophoblast.)

That said, if there is a genuine attempt to transplant an embryo of an appropriate age to be transplanted—an attempt which would require a belief that successful transplantation was not impossible for that embryo—this could be compared with high-risk surgery as a final attempt to save an older patient, for example. As such, removal and transplantation to the uterus would be potentially justifiable if safe for the mother, even in cases where it was more likely to kill than cure the embryo who is otherwise, as Kaczor points out (271), doomed to die (given that survival of an ectopic child to be surgically delivered alive—see note 96 of this chapter— is so rare that it can be practically discounted, unless the pregnancy is discovered when it is already far advanced).

101　Even if we see the placenta as dysfunctional in some way, we should not assume that a dysfunctional, but still-functioning organ—in this case, an organ of the fetus—may be lethally excised. Cutting out the heart of a baby with heart disease would be immoral, even if the heart disease was affecting another person (say, a conjoined twin whose own heart was being dangerously overloaded).

102　Indeed, the 'dead donor' rule for the harvesting of some organs suggests that we believe this even in cases where organ harvesting—though mutilating the person by permanently destroying a level of functionality for that person — does not hasten death, because ventilation has in any case just been withdrawn. Not all mutilation hastens death; for example, the elective removal of healthy eyes is mutilation, even if death is in no way hastened and even if brain damage has made the person already unable to see.

103　See note 87 of this chapter.

104　A similar thought is offered by O. E. Worcester, a female physician writing in 1894:

"I would as soon take a child from its crib and dash its brains out, as to destroy the youngest fetus . . . This is my plea: 'What God hath joined together let not man put asunder,' in the medical profession or elsewhere" (O. E.

Worcester, M.D., "From a Woman Physician: An Open Letter to Dr. W. W. Parker," *Journal of the American Medical Association* 22 [1894]: 599, reprinted in "JAMA 100 Years Ago", *JAMA* 271.15 [1994]: 1208b).

Relevant here may be the following reflections of Alexander Pruss, which, although referring to deliberate killings of unborn children, may also be applicable to deliberate pre-viability removals without the aim of causing death. Note that Pruss is referring to the applicability to the mother-child relationship in general of the mother's acceptance of the permissibility of abortion in some situations.

"It is plausible that the mother's love for her child has to be *unconditional* in order for the child to develop properly, feel accepted and secure. It is of great value for the child to believe that it has and will always be loved unconditionally. And this kind of love not only is incompatible with actually aborting the child, but is incompatible even with deliberating about aborting the child. For mere deliberation about whether there is sufficient reason to abort the child would be an acknowledgment that there *could* be sufficient reason to abort the child, and hence would be incompatible with an unconditional love. If one believes that there *could* be sufficient reason to abort a child, then one cannot rationally have an unconditional love for a child. But, plausibly, the child *needs* such a love. It should not be strange to think that there are some things that it is wrong to deliberate about. If one is, for instance, deliberating whether to practice cannibalism on one's own toddlers one has already done wrong. Some deeds are so horrendous that there is reason not to even deliberate about them, or at least deliberate in the sense of weighing considerations pro and con.

Thus, a mother who thinks that abortion is sometimes acceptable but who chooses not to abort, needs to act irrationally in order to fulfill the needs of her child. She needs to deceive herself into thinking that there cannot be a reason to abort *this* child. A moral view that requires self-deception as a pre-condition for the proper fulfillment of ordinary human functions such as motherhood will be unsatisfactory. Leading the examined life should not be incompatible with leading a genuinely human life" (Pruss, "Maternal Love and Abortion").

105 Garcia, "Intentions in Medical Ethics", 173–4.

106 It may be asked why the acceptance of lethal side-effects for the baby of one's cancer treatment would not also go against unconditional maternal love. In fact we do in practice accept some serious knock-on effects for our loved ones of certain acts or omissions in postnatal situations. While the pregnancy relationship is 'special', it cannot be as different as this from other family relationships. It is implausible, for example, that a woman who rejects very expensive maternal-fetal surgery (where the cost would fall on her) because of her obligations to her born children is failing to love her unborn baby—any more than if she rejected very expensive surgery for one of her born children that would catastrophically affect the prospects of the others.

107 Kaczor, 269. For example, it is wrong to say that 'removing' the baby must be in itself morally neutral since in theory, the baby could be moved to a safer place; this is like saying that sexual intercourse would be acceptable—'that very same act' it might be claimed—if only the woman had consented (see note 88 of this chapter), or that cutting deep into a patient would be acceptable if only the aim of the incision had been to treat the patient's disease.

108 This is a point often missed; for example, by Boonin (*A Defense of Abortion*, 224–7) who does not accept that human beings can be wrongly treated as objects of deliberate attack in circumstances where, if they are *not* deliberately attacked, their deaths will still be (permissibly) causally produced.

109   Damage to the woman's reproductive health caused by removing the tube or tube segment (though see note 97 of this chapter) is of course no more intended than lethal damage to the embryo's health: in both cases, this is a foreseen but unintended side-effect of life-saving treatment for the woman.

110   While rightly decrying early delivery that has the baby's death as its object, Peter Cataldo and T. Murphy Goodwin are on less firm ground when they suggest that "When delivery is delayed in spite of a substantive maternal risk, this delay of delivery becomes **an active medical intervention on behalf of the fetus**" (emphasis added), adding later that "The aggressive treatment strategy of delaying delivery could be refused, since the proportionate benefit to the fetus of living a few more weeks is outweighed by **almost any substantive burden on the mother and the family**" (emphasis added) (Peter J. Cataldo and T. Murphy Goodwin, "Early Induction of Labor", in *Catholic Health Care Ethics: A Manual for Practitioners*, second edition, ed. Edward J. Furton with Peter J. Cataldo and Albert S. Moraczewski [Philadelphia, PA: National Catholic Bioethics Center, 2009], 116, 117).

It is true that delivery several months early is sometimes required for serious maternal and/or fetal indications, while reduced benefit for a terminally ill baby will sometimes have moral relevance. However, it is implausible to claim that 'withdrawing pregnancy support' by *actively delivering the child* can be equated to withdrawing or withholding medical treatment—chemotherapy, say. The comparison is unconvincing, given the fact that pregnancy support is a basic, natural function more akin to breastfeeding, while delivery may involve not only actively caused rupture of fetal membranes but other actively caused hazards for the fetus such as those caused by the woman's contractions (see note 23 of Chapter 2 and note 94 of this chapter).

111   See note 74 of this chapter.

112   Cataldo and Goodwin claim that although the placenta is a product of the fetal genome, "its intimate relationship with maternal tissues and its direct effect on maternal health argue for its consideration as a maternal organ in some senses. Moreover, the placenta is not part of the body by which the individual is identified . . . "(118, note 2). However, one could turn this around and claim (again, incorrectly) that the uterine lining and maternal placenta is 'not part of the mother' because of its 'intimate relationship with fetal tissues and its direct effect on fetal health', not to mention the fact that the uterus 'is not part of the body by which the individual is identified.' Such arguments clearly will not do: the fetal placenta, as opposed to the uterine lining and maternal placenta (see Introduction) is a fetal organ, though one discarded, as the maternal placenta is also discarded when it is no longer needed. For a contrary view to Cataldo and Goodwin's, see Bringman and Shabanowitz, "The Placenta as an Organ of the Fetus".

113   Or viability, were the child in better health. Here as elsewhere (see note 87 of this chapter) the question should, I think, be what kind of intervention would seriously harm even a healthy individual of the relevant age. A seven-month-old baby with a lethal anomaly who will die immediately on delivery does not have an automatic right to an extra two months' gestation, if immediate delivery is indicated for the mother, and if a child without the baby's condition would not be very adversely affected by delivery at that gestational age. What makes delivery fatal is not what happens to the fetal membranes (amniotic sac, etc.) *as such*: these are arguably not harmed, or not seriously harmed, by 'breaking the waters' so close to the normal time of birth. It is rather the harmful effects of separation/expulsion from the mother on other parts of the body of the fetus that are at issue: not parts with the normal fragility of parts

of any baby at an earlier stage (what counts as harm to human beings is often age-relative) but rather parts that are so exceptionally fragile that avoiding lethal side-effects on them may be beyond the call of duty.

114 For supporting references, see Kuebelbeck and Davis, *A Gift of Time*, 37. See also Nancy Valko, "The Case against Premature Induction", *Ethics and Medics* 29.5 (May 2004): 1–2.

115 See Appendix.

4 The Spousal Pregnancy

The image of the pregnant body is as symbolically powerful as it is publicly recognizable. The fecund silhouette is a familiar part of our cultural imagery and visual vocabulary. The public attention paid to the pregnant body is especially interesting because of what it symbolizes: the private, the family. It gestures backward toward the intimacy that created the body's prolific shape as well as forward toward the intimacy shared between mother and infant. There is, then, a peculiar and compelling incongruity in the way in which the pregnant body is regarded within the community. It is a body that is immediately and widely distinguishable for what it ideally represents: personal moments, the creation of a family, the sharing of life and lives.[1]

These profound comments of Julie Piering offer a rich and (we might say) a pregnant introduction to the themes of this chapter. Thus far, we have been looking at responses to existing pregnancy, with limited focus, mostly in the grim context of rape, on how the pregnancy began. In this chapter, we will be looking in more detail at the very different ways in which a pregnancy can begin, and at the significance these different ways may have for parents, children and those about them. The question to explore will be whether, morally speaking, there are better and worse ways to begin a pregnancy—naturally and/or deliberately or otherwise—and if so, what these ways might be. Clearly, this is a very large subject to cover in one chapter, though it would be unwise to complete a book on pregnancy without some discussion of it. To those readers who may already feel that the book has by this stage become a little 'broad-brush,' I can only plead that my aim at this point is less to deal with most or even many counterarguments than to present a positive account of pregnancy, and of some approaches to it.

FETAL REDUCTION

To set the scene, and in stark contrast to Piering's opening image, it may be instructive to look at one less happy and far less common narrative for pregnancy, involving the 'reduction' or selective termination of a twin pregnancy following IVF or similar ARTs (assisted reproductive technologies). Such reductions are often practised with higher-order multiple pregnancies to maximise the chances of the pregnancy remaining—though with some unwillingness to 'reduce' (say) triplet pregnancies to a lower number than twins. However, increasingly, reduction to a singleton pregnancy from either twins or triplets is being carried out on women who wish for social (for example, economic) reasons to ensure that only one baby will survive.

The procedure, which involves a lethal injection to the heart of one fetus (chosen for accessibility, or sometimes for its sex) is disturbing to many health care staff[2]—even those who support reduction and abortion in principle—and, indeed, to the women who go through with the procedure. Here is a comment from one woman who was 14 weeks pregnant when she underwent twin reduction. Jenny is 45, and confides to the *New York Times* interviewer that things would have been different had she and her husband been younger, more financially secure and without grade-school age children. She and her husband intend to tell no one about the reduction, not even close friends or (presumably) the twin selected to be born.[3] Though she and her husband have older children, the twins reduced were conceived with donor eggs, following fertility treatments over a period of six years. On this last point, Jenny makes the following observation:

> If I had conceived these twins naturally, I wouldn't have reduced this pregnancy, because you feel like if there's a natural order, then you don't want to disturb it. But we created this child in such an artificial manner—in a test tube, choosing an egg donor, having the embryo placed in me—and somehow, making a decision about how many to carry seemed to be just another choice. The pregnancy was all so consumerish to begin with, and this became yet another thing we could control.[4]

This is a remarkable comment, bearing out as it does the bold and strongly disputed claims of those who attribute the 'consumerish' attitudes of ART doctors and patients to unborn ART offspring to the 'consumerish' structure of ARTs themselves. After all, procedures like IVF, in which isolated parts from male and female are combined outside the body,[5] *are* normally accompanied by quality control of gametes or at least (and more seriously) living embryos who are graded for immediate use, freezing or disposal. The claim is not so much that it is *impossible* for these embryos to be welcomed unconditionally on production but, rather, that the symbolism inherent in embryo production—its strong resemblance to production of subhuman objects—creates a certain pressure that most parents and 'producers' of the embryos do not, in fact, resist.

'Quality control' and disposal of surplus offspring begins in the petri dish and continues well into the pregnancy for those embryos who are neither frozen nor discarded but are immediately 'used' (i.e., transferred to the body of a woman). As the *New York Times* article reveals, couples who have longed for a baby for years may still be prepared not only to screen for disability but to terminate the life of even a healthy twin baby, on the grounds that twins are—as parents of born twins readily admit—quite a challenging affair.

For some people, what is especially troubling—even shocking—about twin reduction is the *withdrawal* of maternal support that has already been deliberately offered in some shape or form. While pregnancy and conception have a very disturbing character of their own if there was *never* an intention to allow a pregnancy to continue (or to begin—embryos might be conceived for research and/or gestated for their tissue),[6] there is a 'downward slide' and a particular kind of betrayal when some degree of maternal support and protection is offered—even if tentatively, not unconditionally—and is then violently curtailed.

To speak of betrayal is not, it should be emphasized, to judge individual parents who succumb to an alarmingly and, it seems, increasingly atomized, consumerist and egocentric culture.[7] Personal culpability depends on many things and is, in any case, not the issue here: the point is rather about objective failures to honor what is already a real parent-child relationship[8] with strong fiduciary demands. Parents, like other human beings, make serious moral mistakes: it helps no one to see choices in this area alone as somehow beyond moral criticism.[9] The customer is *not* always right—in reproduction as elsewhere.

WANTED CHILDREN

It is often assumed—perhaps not surprisingly—that children conceived via ARTs like IVF will be, not less, but *more* loved and welcomed than those naturally conceived. We can think of the deep desire for children ART couples feel, their commitment to each other and the commitment of the doctors whose care and skill will be employed for months or even years. Indeed, the *New York Times* interviewer herself suggests that twin reduction cases are especially troubling "because twin reduction (unlike abortion) involves selecting one fetus over another, when either one is equally wanted". Note that "wanted" here does *not* mean "accepted unconditionally": clearly, human beings, as well as objects, can be "wanted" intensely and possessively but nonetheless conditionally on their meeting certain requirements, failing which they will be rejected and destroyed. These requirements may relate to internal features such as gender, health or ability and/or to external circumstances,[10] such as whether they are 'just enough' or 'one too many' in their parents' eyes.

What might we be missing out on in conceiving via ARTs? —bearing in mind that, leaving aside the more obvious costs and stresses, almost all couples would far prefer to conceive their children in the usual way if they saw this as feasible for them.[11] Sexual conception—but just what about sexual conception might create a better environment for acceptance? Mutual pleasure, of course—though sex for subfertile couples will often involve anxieties that make it less than fully pleasurable for the couple concerned. But what might even less-than-ideal sex provide in terms of acceptance that ARTs do not? (leaving aside for the moment whether any differences are morally conclusive for the choice to use ARTs).[12]

RECEIVING OR PRODUCING

One thing we might point to is the fact that sex—at least, sex of a minimally respectful, non-instrumentalising kind—is not *just* about conception, even for couples who are positively aiming to conceive. Rather, sex for such a couple has a meaning that concerns their *relationship*, their union on several levels: a meaning of a kind not wholly dependent on the aim to conceive on some particular occasion. There is an important distance between the act itself—albeit linked to conception both biologically and, here, intentionally—and the fertile outcome that may or may not result from that act for that couple.

Sexual conception—for those who do achieve it—gives parents an experience of mutual, concurrent[13] and direct (though partial) causal involvement in the creation of their child. At the same time, it takes place in a context which is social in the uniquely intimate sense which the sexual act already so well expresses. As the kind of loving act it should be, sex refers both socially and biologically to children, although (and this is helpful) far less directly than do ARTs, whose sole rationale is the bid to conceive. Even if sex is 'reproductive' in structure, the immediate act is, or should be, about the couple and their (reproductive-type) relationship, whether they can conceive or are trying to conceive or not. Sex is a joint act of persons, as opposed to scattered acts of persons obtaining and manipulating materials, though often with a relationship in mind. If the manufacture of embryos is indeed 'bad symbolism' for conception, perhaps the self-surrender of intercourse of a certain kind[14]—the mutual giving and receiving of whole bodily persons—might be 'good symbolism' for the 'receiving' of a child whom couples are thus prepared to welcome unconditionally, rather than grade or control. Nor is this just a matter of conventional 'symbols': the act of receiving any future child is not conventionally tied to, but is causally the same act as, the act of receiving the other person.[15] There is a reality here for the couple to grasp: a double good to which their act refers. The couple sexually unite, allowing their gametes to unite, allowing a child to be conceived who is then better placed to be received by the couple as a gift, not graded as the product of a making.

In contrast, ARTs encourage the couple to think of themselves as 'commissioners' of the child-product assembled: separated causally from its coming-to-be, but invited to take, explicitly or by default, owner-type attitudes towards it.[16] On the one hand, the couple, while ultimately empowered to reproduce, are disempowered causally as a couple in the sense that they do not help cause/receive their child *together* but separately supply the raw materials for its 'making.' On the other hand, they are invited to exercise radical control over the child-product—its quality and claim to be gestated or discarded—albeit at a distance and via intermediaries. In a similar way to 'purchasing' a child, 'manufacturing' a child begins the parent-child relationship in a way which has quite different connotations from an act of mutual bodily surrender. Production, like purchase, is in fact a dangerously demeaning way to acquire a child, however powerfully desired, even if some parents do welcome children unconditionally once 'bought' or 'produced'.

Conception is a momentous personal event for all concerned, and as such, is appropriately caused by an interpersonal interaction of a kind reserved to those already bonded, and in that way fitted, to care for such a vulnerable result. This interaction, if it is not, and should not be, too solemn an affair, nonetheless possesses some minimal gravitas supplied by the social meaning of the act—which in turn is closely linked to the power this act sometimes has to cause conception, with all that will entail. Such gravitas and such independent interpersonal meaning is necessarily absent from the series of scattered acts involved in (for example) IVF: the technical piecing together of gametes by IVF doctors, preceded by the harvesting of eggs from the woman, and the man's masturbation, often with the aid of pornography supplied by the clinic. The goal itself is momentous, and the would-be parents may be anxiously devoted to achieving that goal; however, this does not guarantee the appropriateness of their means or their respect for the result. (We might think here of artists who can be anxiously, obsessively caught up in the process of making a painting, while still naturally regarding themselves as free—even bound—to destroy a product which falls short of their desires.)

True, the parents of any child conceived can still do their best to take an attitude of unconditional acceptance towards the child at any point. After all, they went into IVF in the first place with a desire to have a child whom they doubtless wished at least eventually to love and accept unconditionally in true parental fashion. Yet should not those approaching parenthood have all the help they need symbolically—in what their bodies signify and cause—to take this attitude right from the start? Is not sex, in its most committed form, a body-language as far as possible removed from the 'manufacturer's logic' of screening and disposal?[17] And is not manufacture, with these connotations of control and domination, something we should eschew altogether as a means to acquire a child?

By analogy, most of us believe that it is wrong to buy a baby online—particularly if the child is purchased pre-conception so that we cannot see ourselves (rightly or wrongly) as 'rescuing' some existing needy child. For a couple to conceive a child in order to sell it, or pay another couple to do so, would be frowned on even if great efforts were subsequently made to protect the child's well-being. In other words, disrespectful forms of conception which tend inherently to the child's disadvantage cannot, we think, be made respectful by concurrent plans to 'pick up the pieces'.

GOOD ENOUGH PARENTS

We spoke of the gravitas of sex as a means to conception, but paradoxically, one welcome outcome of the sexual pathway is that it can bring some 'lightness' to the advent of conception, whether envisaged or discerned. As one writer puts it, "Inseparably united to sexuality, parenthood recovers an element of joy and light-heartedness, even play, just as sexuality recovers an element of responsibility."[18] Certainly, sexual conception can be culpably reckless, even in the context of fertility enhancement, as when a couple risks a high-order multiple pregnancy after the woman's superovulation. More generally, couples do have some responsibility for asking themselves whether they are able to care adequately for any child they may conceive. However, the exclusive and oppressive focus on conception, for which couples can feel portentously but unparentally responsible, is guarded against by the fact that sex can be perceived to have a raison d'être and a potential dignity of its own,[19] including for those unable to conceive. It is also guarded against by the fact that, ideally, the couple have entered, and signify via further acts of 'consummation', an institution that traditionally exists to promote their interests and those of any children they may have. We will return to this later on.

While supporting unreservedly what she describes as "the ability of women to control their fertility," Josephine Johnston, a medical ethicist interviewed in the *New York Times* article, notes that:

> In an environment where you can have so many choices, you **own the outcome** [emphasis added] in a way that you wouldn't have, had the choices not existed. If reduction didn't exist, women wouldn't worry that by not reducing, they're at fault for making life more difficult for their existing kids. In an odd way, having more choices actually places a much greater burden on women, because we become the creators of our circumstance, whereas, before, we were the recipients of them.[20]

Some of this anxiety and perfectionism is very evident in Jenny's story: she is said to have taken pride in being a good mother to her grade-school age children, and to have felt that "twins would soak up everything she had to give, leaving nothing for her older children. Even the twins would be robbed, because, at best, she could give each one only half of her attention and, she feared, only half of her love." Jenny, we are told, "desperately wanted another child, but not at the risk of becoming a second-rate parent." She is quoted as saying "This is bad, but it's not anywhere as bad as neglecting your child or not giving everything you can to the children you have."

Many parents of multiple children, alive as they are to the challenges and burdens, will be bemused by the naive arithmetic proposed here. Aside from the fact that one twin is surely 'robbed' (to use the article's term) of life itself, while his/her siblings are 'robbed' not of half, but of all the future love of someone very like themselves, there is something odd in Jenny's fear that twins imply a minimal—and seemingly uncontrollable—50 per cent reduction in maternal love. Even if this could be confidently predicted, we should be wary of a parental approach that makes the best (or perceived best) the enemy of the good. This is especially so at a point where the child already exists and needs, not an ideal impossible environment, but a basic level of care that the parent/parents can and should provide.[21] The 'good enough parent' is simply the parent who does what is reasonable in her own circumstances and with her own commitments—including all her children, of any age, number or location. Loyalty demands that she respect the rights of each of those children: rights that will never be to the impossible in terms of love, care and attention from her or from the father, but only to the possible and reasonable. In any case, deliberate lethal bodily invasions of children, born or unborn, can always be avoided: negative rights of this kind can be binding in a way that most positive rights cannot. A frenetic household may be hard to live in, and may justify all manner of stratagems, but lethal reduction is simply not a humane or an equitable way to escape it.

DONOR PREGNANCIES

The situation of Jenny is, of course, complicated by the fact that her twins were conceived with donor eggs, a fact which raises important ethical issues of its own. To begin with, we need to ask: Is Jenny, at 45, infertile, or simply menopausal?[22] If she is infertile, did donor conception *treat* her infertility? Or did it not rather help Jenny's (presumably) fertile husband to conceive children jointly with a younger and more fertile woman, in the form of the egg donor? A woman who took the risks egg harvesting involves, who was almost certainly paid for her trouble,[23] and who was very possibly paid extra for 'high quality' eggs, if she came from some sought-after group (good looking, intelligent, high-achieving).

Jenny, it is true, then *became the mother* of the embryos in the very act of having them transferred to her body: her maternal rights and duties began at that point (or so I have been arguing in this book). However, the *opportunity to exercise* a 'reproductive' ability like gestation *subsequent* to reproduction by another woman does not mean that one has 'reproduced' on one's own account—with assistance or without it. One has 'reproduced', i.e., 'produced' a new human individual only when one is the genetic parent of the child conceived, and this applies here not to Jenny but to the egg donor conceiving with her husband. Is there not something unhealthy about a society where women—even women of 45, even where they have other children, even where they need to use another woman's body—feel drawn to such lengths to have a baby?

We should recall that in the case of surrogacy, commissioning couples are assured by surrogacy brokers and clinics that they are the 'real' parents of the child, while the surrogate is said to be merely a 'carrier.'[24] Here, it is the 'carrier' who is also the commissioner, who receives the message that she is the 'real parent', though the ovum donor is genetically no less linked to the offspring than the woman's husband, if his sperm was used.[25] A husband, moreover, for whom presumably this genetic link with his children was seen as important, and for that reason positively sought. Are not *all* these people parents of a kind—and in that case, can we confidently justify so fragmenting parenthood,[26] before the offspring we fragment it for have even been conceived?[27] Is this not, so to speak, a form of 'one-night stand parenthood'[28] on the donor's part, which should not be invited or pursued, however generous the motive?[29] If for purposes of (e.g.) child support, we count conception via intercourse as giving rise, however unwittingly, to parenthood, surely *deliberate* conception via donation can make those who do this true genetic parents, though the donor is pre-emptively excluded from his/her child's care.[30] Bearing and raising children does promise to bring a very real form of flourishing to couples—but there are many other ways to flourish without the moral cost, if we can call it such, of using donors.

The fact that one would-be social parent is actively seeking the very genetic and social link with the child that is denied the child[31] in relation to the donor has not escaped the attention of those donor offspring who object, as some such offspring do, to their manner of conception. Joanna Rose, who took a court case in Britain resulting in a judgment[32] against anonymous donation of gametes, has strong comments to make on donor conception per se—in her case, via donor sperm. Despite her deep affection for the family she was raised in, and her willingness to understand the (presumably benevolent) motives of the donor thanks to whom she now exists, she regards her pre-planned deprivation of that donor father as inherently unjust:

> Just as infertility is grieved, because people grieve the loss of having and raising their own genetic children, so too can that loss be mirrored by not knowing or being raised by one's own genetic parents. Indeed, for many, this loss is exacerbated when it is intentionally and institutionally created, unlike infertility.[33]

Rose adds that:

> To seek to excuse this by asserting that those so produced should be grateful to be "wanted" and "loved", or even to exist, is a dangerous

way to think and will lead to inevitable and increasing assaults on the identities of future generations. The burden of infertility must not be circumvented by ill-considered quick fixes that pass the baton of grief and loss to the next generation.[34]

Rose is surely right to reject a test for justified conception that looks merely to the value of the existence of those to be conceived. Conceiving a child to be auctioned live on television would result in a life which—arguably, like every human life—has meaning and value.[35] The same applies to (say) deliberately conceiving a child via prostitution or consensual incest. Yet precisely because the child's life *has* a special value, that value should be respected in its bringing into being, in a way we do not feel we need to respect the bringing into being of farm animals, for example. This is a theme explicitly raised by another donor offspring, who comments starkly as follows:

> They created me in the same way as they breed pigs. All I know and am allowed to know about my father is that he masturbated his 'sample' for a sum. Yes you could say I'm angry.[36]

While, clearly, not all donor offspring feel this way, the question is not so much how many feel this way[37] as whether those who *do* feel this way might not perhaps have reasonable grounds. Is donor conception adequate to the bringing into being of new persons? Is it a dignified and respectful process?[38] Some people, including some donor-conceived people—and even some donors and some social parents[39]—believe that it is not.

ACCEPTING DONOR EMBRYOS ('EMBRYO ADOPTION')

The fact that even some social parents come later to regret their use of donors raises the question of what Jenny should have done in the—perhaps unlikely—event she had changed her mind about donation after the creation of the embryos, but before their transfer to her body. The answer might seem obvious, if these are genuine children, albeit very young ones: have them transferred anyway, and become their permanent committed mother. However, is this really the solution? Do not these embryos already have a mother, in the form of the egg donor?[40] In any case, should Jenny be attempting to become their mother in this purely clinical way? While clinical procedures do seem quite acceptable as treatments to help existing mothers nurture children,[41] such procedures are arguably no more adequate as a way of *becoming* a mother, in the absence of any truly interpersonal act, than is IVF itself. Nurture and creation are two very different things; however, starting to nurture in this case does create a new mother, if not new human lives. And while there are injustices involved in the in vitro manufacture of embryos which are not involved in their transfer to an unrelated woman once they exist, we should not assume that embryos and women cannot also be disrespected by such transfer even if it allows the embryos to be safely born. (After all, we might want to say something like that about commercial surrogacy, which we might identify as demeaning women and embryos even if it were the only practical way of bringing the embryos to term.)

Embryo 'adoption' or 'donation' is a controversial issue—even more so indeed than IVF, dividing as it does even IVF opponents.[42] It is true that embryo transfer to an unrelated woman responds to, and does not cause, the plight of embryos outside the body:[43] an important difference, even if their creation was commissioned by the woman to whom they are transferred. However, there is also an important difference between embryo transfer to an unrelated woman—sometimes called 'embryo adoption', a term I will use for convenience to include transfer to an unrelated 'commissioner'[44]—and conventional social adoption of a born child, to which embryo adoption is often compared. For unlike with social adoption, there is with embryo adoption a specific act, transferral to the unrelated woman's body, that can be seen as wrongly supplanting intercourse rather as IVF does, even if not in the same way or to the same extent (it seems rather closer to 'rescuing' the embryos via commercial surrogacy, though the surrogate's motives will of course be different).[45] IVF supplants intercourse in the all-important role of creating the child—not just a mother for the child. However, embryo adoption also, by its very nature, makes a woman a biological mother, with strong and overriding maternal rights and duties, but is nonetheless a 'technical' act with no independent human-spousal meaning of its own.

A keystone of the sexual act from the side of the woman is the woman's psychophysical 'openness' in some sense—not always a literal or practical sense—to becoming a mother via becoming pregnant. It is precisely this openness in the course of an *interpersonal* act between the couple with its own independent meaning that embryo adoption replaces as a means of becoming a biological mother.[46] (As argued in the last chapter, the mere fact of being pregnant suffices to make a woman a mother, with the presumptive right to raise the child. This is in contrast to a woman who has just adopted a child postnatally, who may for some time be morally and legally liable to have the child taken back by a birth mother who has changed her mind.)[47]

We should note that a pregnancy begun by embryo adoption—perhaps with very generous, life-saving motives on the adopting couple's part—will communicate a radically misleading message about the child's origin in a way that has no parallel with couples simply taking their postnatally adopted child out with them in public—or indeed, looking after other people's children.[48] Children are quite easily and naturally looked after from time to time by biologically unrelated adults: there is no single act of looking after children which signifies unequivocal parenthood. In contrast, intercourse creates a state of pregnancy that *does* have that significance waiting to be discovered by the parents and by those about them. Pregnancy, if naturally achieved and left to itself, is a more reliable sign of origin even than breastfeeding, which, again, is easily and (in some cultures) not infrequently provided by those other than the mother. In contrast, embryo adoption turns something—the visible state of pregnancy—which has unique value as a supremely trustworthy sign of origin into a sign of, at most, ongoing parenthood and parenting intentions, not original parental provenance of the child.

As mentioned earlier, embryo adoption is hotly disputed, and there are certainly some less convincing arguments against it, beginning with generic appeals to 'unnaturalness' of a kind that would include morally unexceptionable medical procedures.[49] Such unspecified unnaturalness is of course no better an objection to embryo adoption than it is to IVF, where the real concern is not so much the replacing of missing elements in natural conception but, rather, what exactly is replaced. With intercourse, one and the same interpersonal act unites the couple at several levels and (with or without medical assistance[50]) helps to cause their child to exist if the right conditions obtain. The connection between sex and pregnancy is complicated: a marriage can be consummated, for example, without a pregnancy beginning or having a chance to begin, and even perhaps if subsequent steps were taken to prevent a pregnancy beginning or continuing due to a sudden change of heart.[51] Nonetheless, pregnancy is part of the meaning of intercourse—the further good to which it is tending—even for those who cannot conceive, let alone carry a pregnancy to term. The immediate structure of uncontracepted intercourse is inseparably 'open' to pregnancy and to conception, even if factors outside the couple's control mean that the general 'fertile structure' of the act will not have a 'fertile result'. Those who object to replacing this structure of sexual self-giving with a structure of technical production in the case of IVF need to explain why another 'technical' way of becoming a mother—embryo adoption[52]—is not also a harmful supplanting of a deeply significant interpersonal act as a way of entering on parenthood. If it truly is the case that a woman becomes a mother in becoming pregnant—which, of course, many people will deny—the onus of proof is on those who reject IVF while accepting embryo adoption as a means of becoming a biological mother to show why the latter does not share too much in common with IVF, for all the differences between them.

PREGNANCY, INTIMACY AND SOCIETY

To return to Piering's opening image: what, ideally, would the "intimacy that created the body's prolific shape" involve, on the view I am proposing? To begin with, it would provide the pregnancy with clear and unambiguous information on parentage: not just unambiguous information on maternity (this woman, and she alone, is the mother of this child) but information on paternity (this visibly linked, publicly committed life partner of this visibly pregnant woman, and he alone, is the father of this child). That way, children know who they are and have unrestricted access to parts of their biological and social history that may influence their present and their future; they also avoid being torn emotionally between competing claimants for motherhood or fatherhood.[53] Similarly, those outside the family know who to congratulate, who to warn, who to ask for permission to pick up the baby, feed the toddler and so on. Such public linking encourages the father to be fully involved in parenting his child: to support the child's mother in the 'pregnancy endeavor' and thus to become himself a social parent,[54] and not just a genetic parent, from before the child is born. The man learns his fatherhood not only from the woman—who makes available to him experiences of bonding with the fetus[55]—but from others about him who affirm his fatherhood not only after birth but long before it.[56] The commitment morally required of him is major, so the better prepared he is in all these ways, the better patently for him and, even more obviously, for his co-parent and their child.

How is it possible to retain pregnancy as a completely reliable sign of origin? Most clearly, by linking the onset of pregnancy to sexual acts, and by linking sexual acts exclusively to the kind of permanent, public commitment that best protects the interests both of children and of parents.[57] It should come as no surprise that married biological parents, who have committed themselves to each other, often with children in mind, do better both in avoiding abortion and in bringing up successfully any children born. Being raised by married biological parents does seem to be best for children on several levels, according to a large body of research.[58] Of course, this is not to say that children conceived in less-than-ideal ways cannot be lovingly reared by single parents, usually mothers. Such parents make the best they can of the missing parent's absence, but do not normally regard this themselves as the ideal situation for childrearing. Nor is cohabitation the ideal situation: cohabiting couples are orders of magnitude more likely to split up while their children are young[59]—again, unsurprisingly, as they have made no public commitment not to do so.

Many have written eloquently of the adverse effects of the sexual revolution on women, and in particular, on the poorest women who are disproportionately burdened by a free sexual market. As Helen Alvaré notes:

> If high-volume sexual experience produced tangible benefits for women, we would have seen evidence of this by now. Instead, data about female happiness, sexually transmitted diseases, nonmarital pregnancies, abortion, post-abortion distress, cohabitation and divorce tend to point in the same direction. Women—and by extension their children—are suffering unique harms, with the poorest, most vulnerable groups of women losing the most ground.[60]

Perhaps it is time now to admit, without fear or favor, that there is a better way of doing things: better for women, for children, born or unborn, and also for men, insofar as they too have an interest in close, loving and effective parenting. Marriage creates a protected space in which to procreate and bring up children safely with the father's involvement and ideally that of both extended families. While, of course, infertile people can and do have happy marriages, and the benefits of marriage are in no way limited to the actual achievement of conception, marriage as an institution is traditionally built around parenting, hence its proven success in supporting parents and the children they conceive. And while there are certainly bad marriages, and marriage partners should be wisely chosen, the marriage institution does do some part of the work in, so to speak, 'sorting out the men from the boys' (and the women from the girls), and encouraging a continued wish to commit. Subsequent pregnancies can then represent, to the parents, the child and to wider society, a spousal past, present and (hopefully) a spousal future also.

ACCEPTANCE OF FERTILITY

At this point, the restive reader might, however, ask, not unreasonably, whether a spousal meaning of some kind for pregnancy could not be equally well achieved by reserving, not sex itself, but only fertile sex to marriage: a kind of two-tier sexual system. Does not contraception help us do just that, for those of us who wish to do so? Unfortunately contraception cannot be safely relied on to limit conception only to committed willing couples—and not just because contraception, particularly in its more reversible forms, can and does fail. More controversially, use of contraception can encourage the view that fertility is a bad or tiresome feature of sex— and, more worryingly, the view that the child is an interloper whose presence the parents have actively attempted to prevent, and should therefore not be forced to tolerate.[61] In practice, 'withdrawal' of fertility via contraception (as opposed to accepting and 'working around' the woman's fertile days) often accompanies refusal to accept any offspring who may still be conceived. Increased use of contraception seems often to accompany an increase, and not, as one might expect, a decrease, in the practice of abortion.[62] Even those who accept the use of contraception in principle must acknowledge that a child conceived after *failed* contraception does not come into being in an optimal way, but as part of a body-language of active 'refusal', and not merely of 'avoidance'. An analogy sometimes given is that of actively 'disinviting' someone from a party, rather than simply declining to invite him or her on some occasion or, more tactfully still, arranging the party for a day when he or she is out of town. Alternatively (again, a very imperfect analogy, as unconceived children do not yet exist) we might think of expressions of affection: pushing the loved one away seems to create more of an 'atmosphere of rejection' than keeping one's distance to avoid untimely hugs— say, from a child when the parent is otherwise engaged.

The best way of protecting children's interests in parental welcome and acceptance is, plausibly, simply to protect the spousal-parental meaning of *all* sexual acts, not just those intended to result in a child. This can be done by making those acts quite specific to the child-protective institution of marriage; it can also be done by not deliberately withdrawing the fertility from any of these acts, should such fertility be present, as it will be on some days of a fertile woman's cycle. Such parental meaning as sexual acts have, whether or not they will result in a child, is retained and respected by respecting *both* the spousal-parental institution *and* the acts that celebrate that institution.[63] If sexual acts are left with all their spousal meaning,[64] and with all their fertility at any given time, couples are helped to take full responsibility for those acts and for the lives they may engender. Those who wish to be parentally minded, if only for the sake of future children they may have, can benefit significantly by leaving untouched all parental meaning in all acts in this whole area, so that where conception is not thought appropriate, these acts will be avoided or postponed. We learn by doing, and acceptance of fertility is both entirely possible and extremely useful— useful enough to be morally mandated—in encouraging acceptance of each and every child.

The argument here is not, of course, that couples need be intending conception every time that they make love.[65] The willingness may be more along the lines of openness to a child, rather than a positive intention to conceive one. The word 'open' can mean anything from lack of obstruction (in awareness of the general fact that babies come from sex) right through to using knowledge of the woman's menstrual cycle not to avoid conception but to achieve it.[66]

Importantly, such openness will apply only where the couple are united in an act with its own positive rationale in terms of their union as a 'we', aside from any further aim of conceiving. We would not describe someone as 'open' to conception, or to the other person, if they were viewing the other person as a mere subhuman instrument to produce a pregnancy, as might be the case with rape, for example. And as we saw in the case of ARTs, we would not describe the couple as 'open' to conceiving when the whole point of what they do is uniting their gametes, while they themselves do not unite.

SEXUAL CONCEPTION: OF WHAT KIND?

It will by now be clear that in defending sexual conception as a better preparation for parenthood than ARTs, I am in no way defending sexual conception of no matter what shape or form.[67] There are many damaging, immoral and dangerous ways for children to be naturally conceived: from rape to prostitution to one night stands to extramarital affairs. There are also other, less dramatic, failures of couples to make the kind of full and public commitment to each other that best prepares for parenthood. Many such pregnancies are aborted, so the child conceived is lost for a lifetime—to him or herself, to the parents and to other people. Contraception is often cited as the way to stop this happening, but when it fails, it leaves in practice abortions and fatherless families in its wake. The stakes are high, even if (or rather, because) all lives, however conceived, have value and importance. We should never use that value as an excuse for child-hostile, child-neglectful choices.

In the words of Erika Bachiochi:

> Might there be something awry in a sexual ethic in which the pleasure of adults trumps the life of a human being? And, would we not want to rethink how to properly satisfy the human need for intimacy if such satisfaction, as currently pursued, often ignores the reproductive potential of the sexual act (a biological reality that can never be entirely within our control)?[68]

We began this discussion with Jenny's suggestion that she would not have had selective reduction had her pregnancy been naturally conceived. Of course, many naturally conceived children are in fact, if not reduced, nonetheless aborted or considered for abortion—for example, subjected to prenatal tests with a view to abortion should the baby be disabled. However, we need to ask how many of these 'threatened' conceptions are experienced by uncommitted parents and/or those whom contraception has accustomed to think of fertility—and then of an actual unborn child—as an unwanted (or at best, conditionally wanted) intruder on them and on their lives. If the fetus-as-intruder view should be rejected, as I argued in the second chapter, so too should the 'sperm-as-intruder'[69] or 'female-fertility-as-intruder' view, which is significantly different, but can and does prepare the way for the first view in the couple's mind. If it is wrong to see a new human life as an enemy or some kind of dysfunction, it is also wrong, and makes the first more likely, to see fertility itself—the very presence of fertile body-parts—as an enemy or illness or dysfunction. Neither pregnancy nor fertility more generally is a disease of any kind. That fact should affect not only how we view abortion—which impacts catastrophically on the unborn child—but how we view contraception and sterilisation. The power to bear children is a gift, not a defect of the fertile woman: a gift to be responsibly used, like the corresponding gift of the committed male partner she may choose.

FEMALE AND MALE PARENTHOOD

Pregnancy involves a man not only biologically but morally: he should be 'in it for the long haul'. It is wrong to treat pregnancy as a woman's affair alone, even if there is a real sense in which female parenthood is richer than male parenthood, so that a woman is 'more a parent' to her child than a man. This extends not only to the woman's somewhat greater genetic contribution (women contribute mitochondrial, not just nuclear DNA as part of a very much larger gamete) to the fact that the child lives and (normally and ideally) begins in a physical relationship with the mother in a sense in which he or she is not in a physical relationship with the father. The impoverishment involved in surrogacy and egg donation, if these do indeed fragment parenthood, is possible only because of the particular richness of the parenthood these practices fragment.

MALE SUPPORT OF PREGNANCY

Having said that, it is important to remember the kind of contribution that men can, and normally should, make to their child's gestation and not just its conception. This is a theme explored at some length by Norvin Richards, who comments insightfully as follows:

> Although it is true that parenthood requires nothing of men biologically during pregnancy, it doesn't follow that it requires nothing of any kind. After all, nothing biological is required of fathers *after* a child is born; why couldn't the same be true at this stage? A different thought is that a man cannot act *directly* with regard to a child that is not yet born, but only by way of actions toward the pregnant woman. However, this too would provide no reason to think there is nothing for him to do as a father ... it is certainly part of being a father to intercede on your child's behalf if someone else is mistreating her, even if doing so affects the child only indirectly, through its effects on the other party. Since indirect actions are part of fatherhood after the child is born, they might also be part of it before then.[70]

Richards draws the helpful analogy of music being played by a group of musicians, which remains a mutual project even at times at which one or other player is silent:

> Although parenthood can certainly become a solo act, at this point it is supposed to be a mutual project. This does not mean each party must be active in the project at all times, of course, any more than musicians who are performing a piece together must each be playing at all times ... we need not find that there are any specific acts of fatherhood that all fathers are called upon to perform while their children are *in utero*. In particular, it will be open for couples to define their roles, including arrangements under which one of them is to do nothing at all for a period.[71]

Richards continues:

> Still, the leeway couples have isn't absolute. There are still requirements that derive from the parenthood being a mutual project, and

these would apply to every such relationship. For example, one part of participating in a mutual project is permitting the others to play their parts. . . . Where the mutual project of parenthood is concerned . . . one way for a man to fail to act as a father while a woman is pregnant with his child is to behave in ways he knows (or ought to know) would make it difficult for her to play *her* part . . . withdrawing financial support on which she had relied would ordinarily be one way for a man to act substantially in ways he knew (or should know) would make it difficult for the woman to play her part in what is supposed to be their mutual project. Arguably, then, men who stop paying the bills in such cases have stopped being fathers, because they are not even minimally coordinating their behavior with that of the other party to the mutual project of parenthood. The same would be true of a man who regularly acted in ways likely to cause a miscarriage.[72]

We might take issue with Richards' assertion that a man who acts this way has ceased to be a father, rather than simply being a bad father. Even the total abandonment of the pregnant woman, while it would certainly make him cease to be a *social* father (if indeed he ever was one) cannot make him cease to be a *genetic* father. Many roles can be held badly without one's ceasing to hold them at all: ceasing to care for one's elderly parents, for example, does not make one cease to be their child. However, there is much in what Richards says about the ways that fathers can support prenatally—or, at very least, fail to obstruct prenatally—the parenting endeavor. Richards mentions miscarriage: interestingly, there are ways in which the father of an unborn child can make miscarriage less likely, even before the child is conceived. There is a real biological sense in which, in the words of one commentator, spouses "gestate their embryo together".[73] This happens not only through the basic social support that a caring male partner can provide for the pregnant woman, but from the very fact that monogamous intercourse, before and after conception, can support pregnancy: the more the couple have (or have had) intercourse together, the more the woman's body is prepared immunologically to accept, and not reject, the body of a child who is half hers and half the father's. In its full significance, intercourse encompasses not just conception, but gestation and postnatal nurture, which again is helpfully supported by bonding hormones for both parents, before and after birth.[74] The couple's sexual life looks towards a shared lifetime with each other and their baby or babies: it is not just about pair-bonding but about parenthood; not just about motherhood but about fatherhood; not just about pregnancy but about parenting long-term.

CONCLUSION

Pregnancy stands at the crossroads: a private space that becomes visible and public. Ideally, if relevant norms have been respected—or so I want to claim—it signals back to past commitment of the parents, as well as forward to their further commitment to each other and the life they have conceived. Pregnancy strikingly begins our existence in relationship: sex is the precondition not just for the creation of living human beings but for the immediate, if at first unconscious, nurturing of those human beings. For thousands of years, conception, pregnancy and (natural) parenthood were always coextensive: there was no divorce between a child's origin and his or her origin 'in relation' to the woman who helped bring him or her into being. And for thousands of years, social mores at their most humane, when honestly observed, have protected the child's interest also in the father's involvement in his or her life as a whole, not just its coming to be.

In the words of David Velleman,

> Some truths are so homely as to embarrass the philosopher who ventures to speak them. First comes love, then comes marriage, and then the proverbial baby carriage. Well, it's not such a ridiculous way of doing things, is it? The baby in that carriage has an inborn nature that joins together the natures of two adults. If those two adults are joined by love into a stable relationship—call it marriage—then they will be naturally prepared to care for it with sympathetic understanding, and to show it how to recognize and reconcile some of the qualities within itself. A child naturally comes to feel at home with itself and at home in the world by growing up in its own family.[75]

How many children are born and raised in this way? Thankfully (for those of us on a similar wavelength here to Velleman), still millions worldwide. Millions of children know where they come from—which helps them understand where they are going. Genetic and gestational parenthood have value in themselves, and they help prepare for social parenthood. And while the parental meaning of pregnancy has perhaps never been so obscured as it has recently become, there is, I have tried to show, one objective feature of pregnancy which no amount of parental confusion is able to destroy. It is, moreover, a feature which is, in fact, still frequently retained in the consciousness of many pregnant women and girls, even in the most desperate situations. In the words of one woman, a former drug-abusing teenager whose pregnancy she believes saved her life, "I didn't know who the father was. But I knew who the mother was."

Pregnancy is both an aspect of, and a powerful symbol for, the fact that we all begin 'in relationship'.[76] It is the age-old way in which a child's presence is created, and then signalled to the world. The value of pregnancy is there immediately: it does not have to be 'injected in' from without.[77] Having said that, the woman can indeed confer, as well as finding, meaning in her pregnancy, just as in her relationship with the child when it is born. The parent-child relationship concerns objective needs, and calls objectively for certain attitudes, but every parent's experience of this relationship will be different—and that is often a good thing.

Pregnancy tests our commitment, if such we have, to human equality, and to the bodily nature of human moral subjects. It involves a connection of two living, bodily beings, which is normally functional rather than dysfunctional, and which it takes a violent act or some dysfunction to sever. It can be burdensome—even very burdensome—but is not an illness in itself. Pregnancy is maternal: it involves basic maternal support for a dependent child. We should take seriously the fact that we have two subjects here, whose relationship may be more, but is certainly not less, familial than that of other human beings. Let us celebrate pregnancy, then, as a unique and richly meaningful process for ushering in the next generation, and support the women and men who make this possible in every way we can. That very much includes those for whom pregnancy is not a happy event, and who feel alone and unsupported. While there is much to improve in regard to respect for women, their fertility and the children they bear,[78] we should not lose sight of the joy of having children—children seen as a gift, not a product—as we support each other through the obstacles that may cloud or obviate that joy.

NOTES

1 Julie Piering, "The Pregnant Body as a Public Body," 178. Cf. Rothman: "We have in every pregnant woman the living proof that individuals do not enter the world as autonomous, atomistic, isolated beings, but begin socially, begin connected. And we have in every pregnant woman a walking contradiction to the segmentation of our lives: pregnancy does not permit it. In pregnancy the private self, the sexual, familial self, announces itself wherever we go. Motherhood is the embodied challenge to liberal philosophy, and that, I fear, is why a society founded on and committed to liberal philosophical principles cannot deal well with motherhood" (Rothman, *Recreating Motherhood*, 59).

2 Ruth Padawer, "The Two-Minus-One Pregnancy", *New York Times*, August 10, 2011, http://www.nytimes.com/2011/08/14/magazine/the-two-minus-one-pregnancy.html?pagewanted=all; see also Liza Mundy, "Too Much to Carry?", *Washington Post*, May 20, 2007, http://www.washingtonpost.com/wpdyn/content/article/2007/05/15/AR2007051501730.html.

3 It should not be assumed that the surviving twin will not discover—or at least be affected by—the loss of his/her sibling: see the website www.wombtwin.com for personal accounts from twins surviving the prenatal death of siblings. On psychological issues raised by fetal reduction for parents and surviving siblings, see Elizabeth Bryan, "Loss in Higher Multipregnancy and Multifetal Pregnancy Reduction", *Twin Research* 5 (2002): 169–74.

4 Padawer, "The Two-Minus-One Pregnancy".

5 Even ARTs that take place inside the woman's body—for example, artificial insemination (AI)—may involve selection of, e.g., donor sperm (from an intelligent donor, or one who resembles the intended father) as well as a mechanical procedure to inseminate it. Moreover, AI is still an interaction between persons, tools and gametes, not directly between persons. That said, there is one element of 'bad symbolism' AI lacks: the need, as in IVF, to make a separate choice to have the embryo transferred to the woman after its isolated,

'homeless' conception. With IVF the embryo does not begin 'in relationship' to its mother in the most basic bodily sense—let alone the richest human/spousal sense.

6   Deliberate conception to produce a fetus who will then be aborted for its tissue is defended by, among others, John Harris (*Wonderwoman and Superman: The Ethics of Human Biotechnology* [Oxford: Oxford University Press,1992], 110, 129–31).

7   As one recent commentary notes, "Abortion is both a symptom of the breakdown of social bonds, and a cause of further disintegration of the support networks that sustain the vulnerable" (Wolf-Devine and Devine, "A Communitarian Pro-Life Perspective", 65). See also Colombetti, "Relazione e desomatizzazione", 199).

8   More generally, I would argue, it is a failure to honor the right of an innocent human being to immunity from lethal assault—whether from the parents, the doctor or anyone else.

9   There is a strong taboo in some social circles concerning criticism of other people's choices in the area of continuing or terminating pregnancy. However, it is illogical to see this important area of life as in some way immune from moral scrutiny: compare childrearing, which we *are* prepared to criticize both in others and in ourselves.

10   Although fetal anomalies themselves are, of course, internal to the unborn child, parental tolerance or intolerance of those anomalies is an external circumstance of a kind that can and does change.

11   In fact, it is often possible for subfertile couples to achieve conception sexually, albeit with medical assistance—for example, using the approach of NaProTechnology, which closely tracks menstrual cycles and gives targeted treatment as needed. See Joseph B. Stanford, Tracey A. Parnell, and Phil C. Boyle, "Outcomes from Treatment of Infertility with Natural Procreative Technology in an Irish General Practice", *Journal of the American Board of Family Medicine* 21 (2008): 375–84; Elizabeth Tham, Karen Schliep, and Joseph Stanford, "Natural Procreative Technology for Infertility and Recurrent Miscarriage: Outcomes in a Canadian Family Practice", *Canadian Family Physician* 58 (2012): E267–74.

12   Many would accept that sexual conception has a special value; see for example Bertha Alvarez Manninen, who comments: "Human fetuses are created by an act that, ideally, is a physical manifestation of intense love and connection between two human beings. Human fetuses, therefore, are intimately connected to human sexuality, childbearing, and childrearing; they are connected, by their very nature, to other values that we, as a society, hold dear" (Bertha Alvarez Manninen, "The Pro-Choice Pro-Lifer: Battling the False Dichotomy", in *Coming to Life: Philosophies of Pregnancy, Childbirth, and Mothering*, eds. Sarah LaChance Adams and Caroline R. Lundquist [New York: Fordham University Press, 2013], 175–6).

13   Though sex itself is a joint act of persons, the woman's body subsequently facilitates the journey of the sperm to the ovum, by which point the potential father is no longer physically involved. In the case of *in vivo* sexual conception, the woman's immediate physical relationship with the embryo will predate the man's by many months.

14   Pruss, *One Body*; see also Helen Watt (ed.), *Fertility and Gender* (Oxford: Anscombe Bioethics Centre, 2011).

15   Contrast this with receiving, as with (say) artificial insemination, a mere bodily product of someone who need not be even in the room.

16   A former IVF doctor makes the following observations on IVF and parental attitudes:

"Every child is a gift from God. However, the process that brought them into existence has led to an attitude towards the embryo that is no different than any other commodity.

If you add pre-implantation diagnosis into the equation, then you really have a situation that is no different than an auto dealership or a department store. "I will take two of these and then freeze these and toss these." The very people who are showing off their beautiful children will not answer questions about how many frozen embryos are still present or how many they asked to be destroyed.

Also, I doubt that anyone has ever thought how they might describe these things to their children—the fate of their siblings—because they are not seen as such. They are seen as simply a means to an end" ("An IVF doctor has a change of heart", *MercatorNet*, 19 April 2012, http://www.mercatornet.com/articles/view/charge_of_heart).

This last comment seems, however, an overstatement: as noted in Chapter 1, IVF parents may indeed have qualms about their frozen embryos and they may express at least some level of unease about them. Attitudes vary from a determination to have all remaining embryos transferred to the mother to an unwillingness even to engage with the IVF clinic on the subject of their fate. Many parents are equivocal about their embryos' status, in a way that may owe something to feelings of moral discomfort, as the following comment from one IVF mother seems to indicate:

"Little lives, that's how I thought about them. But you have to switch gears and think, 'They're not lives, they're cells. They're science.' That's kind of what I had to switch to" (Munday, "Souls on Ice").

On similar conflicts that may be experienced by health professionals and scientists, see Kathryn Ehrich, Clare Williams and Bobbie Farsides, "The embryo as moral work object: PGD/IVF staff views and experiences", *Sociology of Health and Illness* 30.5 (2008): 772–87.

17 The parents may well be having sexual relations at other times in a way that binds them together as a couple; this does not, however, cancel the 'production' connotations of the means by which their child is actually conceived.

18 Patrick M. Fleming, Review of *The Dignity of Human Procreation and Reproductive Technologies: Anthropological and Ethical Aspects*, *Humanum* (Summer 2012), http://www.humanumreview.com/articles/view/pontifical-academy-for-life-dignity-of-human-procreation.

19 By 'dignity,' I mean moral claim on our respect (see below, including note 38, on 'undignified' forms of conception outside the sexual realm, though of course, some forms of sexual conception can lack moral dignity too).

20 Josephine Johnston, in "Two into One". Johnston does not distinguish between ways of achieving a desired reproductive outcome that may mean very different things in terms of attitudes to children. To delay attempting sexual conception on the ground that one has over-responded to fertility drugs and might conceive twins, triplets etc. might involve a behavioral pattern of avoidance-or-receptivity differing markedly from ART manufacture-and-selection.

21 Prior to conception, there are indeed some ways in which future pressures for parents can be avoided (see below, note 11 above and note 65 of Chapter 3) without going below the 'moral minimum' in terms of respect for one's children, and for the means by which they are conceived.

22 Robert Sparrow's comments on male pregnancy, albeit made from a strongly libertarian perspective, may be apposite here:

"One's sense of the nature and magnitude of [the harms of infertility] depends on an understanding of the role that reproduction and pregnancy play in a normal human life cycle, the joys that they can bring, and the frustrations and suffering of couples who are unable to reproduce and of women who are unable to become pregnant. The moral weight of these frustrations depends on one's knowing that these experiences are central experiences in a normal human life, such that it is appropriate for individuals to regret it deeply when they are unable to experience them.

However, it is simply not the case that pregnancy is a normal part of men's lives. It is not a tragedy when a man cannot become pregnant—no matter how much he wishes to be pregnant" (Robert Sparrow, "Is It 'Every Man's Right to Have Babies If He Wants Them'? Male Pregnancy and the Limits of Reproductive Liberty", *Kennedy Institute of Ethics Journal* 18.3 (2008): 286.

Something similar might, perhaps, be said of a postmenopausal woman who wishes to become pregnant with another woman's externally conceived genetic child. Sparrow's points in regard to male pregnancy are well taken, and can also be applied to some extent to women who use their remaining natural powers—powers not shared by men—to gestate, though without having previously conceived.

Even a woman who is clearly infertile, and for whom the lack of children is a genuine deprivation, is not *helped to reproduce* by egg donation, but is rather *given an opportunity to gestate* an unborn child who originally belongs elsewhere with its first, genetic mother. The 'treatment' the infertile woman receives is less like treatment to ovulate than it is like 'treatment' to enable a woman to breastfeed a baby she wishes to adopt. That said, once the infertile woman is pregnant, we can talk about the healthy exercise of the 'reproductive' function of gestation—even though she has not, in fact, reproduced.

23 This is one reason that some 'donor offspring' object to the use of the word 'donor'—which also has connotations of blood and tissue donation, i.e., acts of uncontroversial benevolence where what is donated has no parental role.

24 John Ozolins comments insightfully as follows:

"The surrogate does not just bear a child, but the child who is to be in an intimate relationship with the commissioning couple (that is, the couple seeking and arranging the surrogacy, irrespective of whether it is a commercial arrangement or not). The child is in an intimate relationship with the surrogate and so also is the surrogate with the infertile couple. This suggests that the exclusive relationship between the commissioning couple is no longer so, since there is another intimately involved in the having of their child. This involvement is different from any other individual who might be said to have a relationship with the couple, since the involvement is directly with what is the most intimate expression of their love . . . The desire to have a child of "one's own" is a couple's desire to embody, out of the conjugal union of their separate bodies, a child who is flesh of their separate flesh made one. This is a very powerful image: the notion that a child is produced through the union of a man and woman who have determined that this is the way in which they will express their love for one another. It is a means of making their love incarnate. Surrogacy cuts across this, even though in the case of gestational surrogacy the child is the genetic offspring of the infertile couple. There does not seem to be any easy way to determine which of the two contributors should be considered the mother—the woman who supplies the ovum or the woman who carries the child. Both have a claim to being the mother of the child. If neither claim can be dismissed, then surrogacy by its very nature must involve three people and so either the notion of an exclusive bond between a husband and wife is destroyed or if this is to be preserved, then the surrogate has to be treated as a commodity . . . this solution seems to be at odds with the very reasons why infertile couples seek treatment for their infertility—they are not seeking extra partners in their relationship" (John Ozolins, "Surrogacy: Exploitation or Violation of Intimacy?" http://www.bu.edu/wcp/Papers/OApp/OAppOzol. htm, 3–5).

25   Sometimes, of course, donor sperm as well as donor eggs will be used, putting the recipient woman in a biologically intimate relationship—a quasi-spousal relationship, in the case of the genetic father—with not just one but two genetic parents. Indeed, perhaps more than two: it is not unknown for embryos from more than one pair of genetic parents to be transferred simultaneously to one woman. Her pregnancy will then communicate seriously misleading information on her babies' origin, while concealing as many as four people who are nonetheless intimately, parentally involved—again, quasi-spousally, in the case of the two fathers—in the children's conception and gestation.

26   Note that genetic parenthood can itself be fragmented, as where an enucleated ovum is given the nucleus of another ovum, and the reconstructed ovum, containing the original 'mitochondrial' DNA outside the cell nucleus, together with the transplanted nuclear DNA, is then fertilized to create an embryo. This technique is proposed to avoid the transmission of mitochondrial disease while retaining a genetic link with the child conceived—who will also, however, have some genetic link with the enucleated egg provider, hence the term 'three-parent IVF'. An alternative technique to which this term is also (wrongly) applied involves, not the *fragmentation* but the *obviation* of genetic parenthood: in this technique, two IVF embryos are destroyed in the process of cloning a new, third embryo from the commissioning couple's embryo, using the second, enucleated 'donor' embryo to provide the bulk of the new embryo, minus the nuclear DNA. On ethical aspects of the two techniques, see the Anscombe Bioethics Centre briefing *Clones and Three-Parent Babies: The Ethics of Mitochondrial Replacement*, http://www.bioethics.org.uk/images/user/ MitochondrialReplacementBriefing14November2012; for a much earlier paper on the first approach, see Helen Watt, "Germ-line Therapy for Mitochondrial Disease: Some Ethical Objections", *Cambridge Quarterly of Healthcare Ethics* 8 (1999): 88–96.

27   As David Velleman rightly observes:
    "That this child cannot be parented by one or both of its biological parents is not a disadvantage that its custodial parents volunteer to mitigate; it was a desideratum that guided them in creating the child, to begin with. Not being attached to a partner with whom they could be fertile, they needed a child who was correlatively unattached, a child already disowned by at least one of its biological parents. Rather than adopt a child whose ties to its biological parents had been ruptured after conception, they intentionally created one for whom those ties were ruptured antecedently. This choice would be morally problematic if biological ties were genuinely meaningful. Hence the need for an ideology that denies their meaning" (J. David Velleman, "Family History", *Philosophical Papers* 34.3 [2005]: 361).

28   Note that although some sequelae of conception can be fairly uncontroversially omitted (breastfeeding, for example, or vaginal birth, for those who need cesarians), to omit childrearing by a premeditated choice to hand the child over to others is to omit a large part of the point of the whole parenting enterprise. As Alexander Pruss has argued, the parental responsibility is not just to 'see to it' that children are cared for by someone, but to do the caring oneself: "It is not just my responsibility to ensure that my children are cared for; it is my responsibility that *I* care for and educate my children, and no one but I can fulfil this responsibility. By ensuring that someone else cares for and educates

my children, the responsibility that my children be cared for is perhaps fulfilled. But the second responsibility is not, since another's care is not my care, except . . . in cases of continuing friendship or other close cooperation. But these cases are not what happens in typical instances of gamete donation. A stranger cannot do *my* caring for and educating of my children, for then it is not *my* caring and educating, but the stranger's" (Pruss, *One Body*, 389–90). Pruss, does not, of course, deny that subsequent to birth it may be necessary to give up a child for adoption, not least for the sake of the child.

29 We would not, after all, approve of a couple who 'donated' their newborn baby to childless dinner guests who looked longingly at the baby—much less a couple who deliberately conceived their first pregnancy with the aim of handing over the child to others (Pruss, *One Body*, 390–2).

30 It is worth remembering that gamete donors will often in fact be conceiving offspring destined not to be raised by others but to be left frozen indefinitely or discarded in the near or distant future. Many IVF embryos are permanently denied any chance of going to term.

31 As David Velleman notes:
"Human families are disrupted in various ways, by death or divorce or poverty or social upheavals. In these circumstances a child is entitled to be raised by parental figures who love it and love one another, even if they are not its biological parents . . . To acknowledge that adopted children have missed something of human importance is not to disparage the children, their parents, or the love and mutual care among them. Similarly, we should not have to disparage anyone in order to acknowledge that the offspring of donated gametes will miss something important as well. And then the contrast between these cases—between compensating children for something they have already lost and creating children with the intention that they never have it—should lead us to question the morality of anonymous genetic donation . . . having a biologically related child is of genuine value, as a potential source of self-knowledge for the parent" (Velleman, "Family History", 371).

For a more skeptical account, which somewhat downplays the objective side of genetic relatedness as a source of potential rights and duties (acknowledged or otherwise), see Hallvard Lillehammer, "Who Cares Where You Come From? Cultivating Virtues of Indifference", in *Relatedness in Assisted Reproduction: Families, Origins and Identities*, eds. Tabitha Freeman, Susanna Graham, Fatemeh Ebtehaj, and Martin Richards (Cambridge: Cambridge University Press, 2014), 97–112.

32 Rose and Another v. Secretary of State for Health and Human Fertilisation and Embryology Authority (2002) WHC 1593.

33 Joanna Rose, "Kinship: Are Some More Equal Than Others?" in Alexina McWhinnie et al., *Who Am I: Experiences of Donor Conception* (Leamington Spa: Idreos Education Trust, 2006): 9. Another donor-conceived offspring comments, "It's hypocritical of parents and medical professionals to assume that biological roots won't matter to the 'products' of the cryobanks' service, when the longing for a biological relationship is what brings customers to the banks in the first place" (Katrina Clark, "My Father Was an Anonymous Sperm Donor", *Washington Post*, December 7, 2006, http://www.washington post.com/wp-dyn/content/article/2006/12/15/AR2006121501820.html).

34 Rose, "Kinship", 9. In the same book, another contributor expresses her opposition not only to her alienation from her donor father but to the non-sexual nature of her origin, which she contrasts with "the serendipitous nature of normal human reproduction, where babies are the natural progression of mutually fulfilling adult relationships" (Christine Whipp, "Worrying the

Wound: The Hidden Scars of Donor Conception", in Alexina McWhinnie et al., *Who Am I: Experiences of Donor Conception* (Leamington Spa: Idreos Education Trust, 2006), 19). Christine Whipp attributes her own very difficult relationship with her mother to the way her mother "related to me as an acquisition"—in Whipp's view, as a direct result of the donor insemination process (24).

35   See Watt, "Life and Health: A Value in Itself for Human Beings?"

36   McWhinnie et al., *Who Am I?* 52.

37   Many studies concerning donor-conceived offspring relate to young or school-age children, while those involving adult donor-conceived offspring are more rare. One very large, albeit non peer-reviewed, study found that adult donor offspring had mixed reactions—including some quite negative reactions—to their origin and were doing less well in several areas than the comparison groups: those raised by biological parents and adoptees (the latter group were admittedly less likely than the donor-conceived to have been told late of their origin). The study authors comment:
"For some donor offspring, the very deliberateness or "intention" with which they were separated, before their birth, from a biological parent is precisely the problem. Moreover, the one group of young people in our study whose conceptions were 100 percent fully intended—that is, the donor offspring—is the same group who, on the whole, are reporting more negative outcomes and experiences of loss, hurt, and confusion. Contrary to the arguments put forth by legal scholars who advocate for a guiding principle based on "intentional parenthood", there is not much empirical basis to suggest that "intentional parenthood" is good for children, and there are substantial reasons to question that principle" (Elizabeth Marquardt, Norval D. Glenn, and Karen Clark, *My Daddy's Name Is Donor: A New Study of Young Adults Conceived through Sperm Donation* [New York: Commission on Parenthood's Future, 2010], 77).
This study has aroused some controversy: for discussion, critique and responses, see the website www.familyscholars.org. Peer-reviewed studies include A.J. Turner and A. Coyle, "What Does It Mean to Be a Donor Offspring? The Identity Experiences of Adults Conceived by Donor Insemination and the Implications for Counselling and Therapy", *Human Reproduction* 15 (2000): 2041–51; A. McWhinnie, "Gamete Donation and Anonymity: Should Offspring from Donated Gametes Continue to Be Denied Knowledge of Their Origins and Antecedents?" *Human Reproduction* 16 (2001): 807–17; V. Jadva, T. Freeman, W. Kramer, and S. Golombok, "The Experiences of Adolescents and Adults Conceived by Sperm Donation: Comparisons by Age of Disclosure and Family Type", *Human Reproduction* 24.8 (2009): 1909–19; Patricia P. Mahlstedt, Kathleen LaBounty, and William Thomas Kennedy, "The Views of Adult Offspring of Sperm Donation: Essential Feedback for the Development of Ethical Guidelines with the Practice of Assisted Reproductive Technology in the United States", *Fertility and Sterility* 93.7 (2010): 2236–46; D.R. Beeson, P.K. Jennings, and W. Kramer, "Offspring Searching for Their Sperm Donors: How Family Type Shapes the Process", *Human Reproduction* 26.9 (2011): 2415–24.

38   For an expression of repulsion on the part of a woman inseminating herself in order to become a surrogate mother, see the comments of Sarah Fletcher: "I agreed to have their baby. I inseminated myself with Mark's sperm, by syringe in my own home. It was an unpleasant and unnatural process but it had to be done. Of course, Mark was not present, but I still felt as if a stranger had invaded my body. I had not realised I would feel this revulsion. For a

moment I thought: "Why am I doing this?" Luckily, I fell pregnant after this first attempt"(Hardy, "Sarah Fletcher has a vocation", 10). Of course, we need to distinguish what may be seen, perhaps inchoately, as *morally* repulsive and undignified—unbefitting the respect due to human conception—from what is seen as undignified in some other way.

39 For testimonies from various perspectives from recipient parents and donors, as well as donor-conceived offspring, see http://anonymousus.org/

40 The egg donor, were she to be approached on this question, would almost certainly decline to gestate the embryos, raising the troubling question of what should then be done with them. They could be kept frozen indefinitely, or perhaps they could be unfrozen on the grounds that this is 'extraordinary' life-support which, though not particularly costly in financial terms, is insufficiently beneficial given that the embryos are prevented from all activity, while nothing can be done morally to help them go to term. The aim in unfreezing the embryos need not be (though in practice it often would be) to hasten their deaths. On the contrary, any willed destruction by passive (or by active) means could be avoided, even if the embryos' deaths are clearly foreseen.

Some have argued that frozen embryos should at least be unfrozen in a way that permits them to resume their activity in an ambience somewhat closer to their natural environment before they would inevitably expire (Nicholas Tonti-Filippini, "The Embryo Rescue Debate: Impregnating Women, Ectogenesis, and Restoration from Suspended Animation", in *Human Embryo Adoption: Biotechnology, Marriage, and the Right to Life*, eds. T.V. Berg and E.J. Furton [Philadelphia and Thornwood: National Catholic Bioethics Center and Westchester Institute for Ethics and the Human Person, 2006], 111–2). The petri dish would act as a kind of artificial womb or fallopian tube—though not, of course, one which could support the embryos more than very briefly. The mother's role is not supplanted here in the way that it would be supplanted by transferral to another woman (or worse, to a man, or to an animal) since the embryos have already been conceived and since a petri-dish is not a parent or pseudoparent of any kind.

The development of real artificial wombs that could support a baby for many months would in practice involve embryo experimentation and effective complicity with IVF practitioners—at least if it did not merely 'work backwards' in improving the incubators that currently support premature babies. In the latter case, it might indeed be a positive development, as a means of saving babies' lives, bearing in mind the fact that the child has begun appropriately in the body of its mother, while a non-personal, non-animal tool for 'gestation' or nurture is not a pseudoparent. In contrast, for women to make use of artificial wombs electively throughout gestation, simply in preference to gestating their own children (Smajdor, "The Moral Imperative for Ectogenesis") would be for them to deprive themselves and the child of a bond of non-trivial importance to their later relationship and to the child's self-esteem and social identity.

41 Embryo transfer could even be attempted to 'rescue' an embryo removed from an ectopic site and allow it to implant in the mother's womb (see note 100 of Chapter 3).

42 For more on these issues, see Sarah-Vaughan Brakman and Darlene Fozard Weaver (eds.), *The Ethics of Embryo Adoption and the Catholic Tradition* (Villanova, PA: Springer, 2007); T.V. Berg and E.J. Furton (eds.), *Human Embryo Adoption: Biotechnology, Marriage, and the Right to Life* (Philadelphia and Thornwood: National Catholic Bioethics Center and Westchester Institute for Ethics and the Human Person, 2006). Having formerly supported

embryo adoption, I argue against it in a paper in *Human Embryo Adoption*, "Becoming Pregnant or Becoming a Mother? Embryo Transfer With and Without a Prior Maternal Relationship". See also Mary Geach, "Motherhood, IVF and Sexual Ethics", in *Fertility and Gender: Issues in Reproductive and Sexual Ethics*, ed. Helen Watt (Oxford: Anscombe Bioethics Centre, 2011), 169–83. See Appendix.

43 This plight does not prove that embryo adoption is legitimate, any more than a patient's need for organs legitimates stealing organs from another person. To 'let someone die' simply because one cannot morally do otherwise is not the same as *intending* that she die.

44 The term is normally restricted to situations where the embryo is transferred to a woman who is neither its genetic mother nor commissioned its production, but intends to raise it as her child.

45 There are degrees of unsuitability here: as we saw earlier, donor insemination does not include *all* the bad aspects of IVF (see note 5 of this chapter), while embryo adoption includes even fewer, since the child already exists.

46 Watt, "Becoming Pregnant, or Becoming a Mother?"; Geach, "Motherhood, IVF and Sexual Ethics".

47 The genetic mother could not, for example, demand the return of her child once transferred (for example, via 'womb flushing' or, less riskily, after the child had been born). In contrast, there is normally and appropriately a cool-off period with postnatal adoption where a birth mother can reclaim the child before the adoptive parents have fully 'grown into' their new rights. Here again, pregnancy creates uniquely strong rights for gestational mother and child to stay together. Pregnancy is not just another form of childcare, to be handed on as and when convenient or requested: it has a special function (as does genetic parenthood) in promoting bonding, the child's sense of identity and the social 'placing' of the child. Bonding is particularly important at the start of the parent-child relationship, and is facilitated by the pregnant woman seeing herself as inextricably bound to the child (as the previous chapter argued) and not replaceable by another woman in her current role.

48 Breastfeeding by those other than the mother is still practised in some parts of the world, and is an easy and natural response in any part of the world where there is a hungry infant—perhaps awaiting its mother's delayed return—and a lactating non-maternal carer.

49 Brandon P. Brown and Jason T. Eberl, "Ethical Considerations in Defense of Embryo Adoption", in *The Ethics of Embryo Adoption and the Catholic Tradition*, eds. Sarah-Vaughan Brakman and Darlene Fozard Weaver (Villanova, PA: Springer, 2007), 107–108. For a discussion of fertility treatments that might fall into this category, see Watt, *Fertility and Gender*, especially the chapters by Mary Geach, Kevin Flannery and Helen Watt. Brown and Eberl also query a claim of Nicholas Tonti-Filippini—surely not intended literally—that pregnancy creates an 'ontological' change in the pregnant woman, which of course cannot literally be the case (108–110).

50 See note 11 of this chapter.

51 Christopher Tollefsen, "Could Human Embryo Transfer Be Intrinsically Immoral", in *The Ethics of Embryo Adoption and the Catholic Tradition*, eds. Sarah-Vaughan Brakman and Darlene Fozard Weaver (Villanova, PA: Springer, 2007), 94. Tollefsen appears to be considering an abortifacient, post-fertilization effect of some drug, rather than a pre-fertilization effect. While Tollefsen does not support such efforts to prevent implantation, I would take issue with his suggestion (96) that the pre-implantation mother-child relationship does not strictly speaking constitute pregnancy, and would appeal to the

coordinated activity of mother and embryo while the embryo is still mobile before its mutually-achieved implantation (see Introduction).

52 To return to a theme of the previous chapter, the fact that the woman to whom the embryos are transferred was not previously the mother is not a 'mere' circumstance of the transfer.

53 Velleman, "Family History".

54 Similarly, it is possible that the husband or partner of a surrogate mother could become a social father via such support, acquiring, as the surrogate herself has acquired via gestation, the right to parent the baby after birth.

55 "It is with mothers, of course, that fetuses have the most direct relationship. And it is on mothers that fetuses have the most direct effects: when they move, the mother feels it. But it is not only to mothers that fetuses relate. The movement of the fetus within is also felt by people in physically intimate contact with the mother, especially her lover and other children. The closer—literally, physically closer—other people are to the mother the closer they are physically and socially to the fetus. When they hold the woman close, they too feel the fetus within. It reaches out to them, and that too is a social experience" (Rothman, *Recreating Motherhood*, 103).

56 Ideally, of course, the man will have had some adequate preparation for fatherhood long before his child was conceived, beginning with his upbringing by his own parents and exposure to good male role models in and outside the family. Like the woman, he is in any case oriented to parenthood *ab initio* by his very physiology, long before any actual parental role he may acquire (what path in life people take and their vocation does not affect this bodily parental orientation).

57 See, e.g., Pruss, *One Body*; Anthony McCarthy, "Marriage and Meaning", in *Fertility and Gender: Issues in Reproductive and Sexual Ethics*, ed. Helen Watt (Oxford: Anscombe Bioethics Centre, 2011); Anthony McCarthy, *Ethical Sex: Sexual Choices and Their Nature and Meaning*, forthcoming.

58 See, e.g., Kristin Anderson Moore, Susan M. Jekielek, and Carol Emig, *Marriage from a Child's Perspective: How Does Family Structure Affect Children and What Can We Do about IT?* Child Trends Research Brief, June 2002; Mary Parke, *Are Married Parents Really Better for Children? What Research Says About the Effects of Family Structure on Child Well-Being* (Washington, DC: Center for Law and Social Policy, 2003); Wendy D. Manning and Kathleen A. Lamb, "Adolescent Well-Being in Cohabiting, Married, & Single Parent Families," *Journal of Marriage and Family* 65 (2003): 876–93.

59 In Britain, the last census found that 97 per cent of all couples remaining together throughout their child's minority were married. Only 3 per cent were cohabiting (Centre for Social Justice, *Response: Child Poverty and Improving Life Chances*, 18 February 2011, http://www.centreforsocialjustice.org.uk/publications/response-child-poverty-and-improving-life-chances).

60 Helen Alvaré, "Abortion, Sexual Markets and the Law," in *Persons, Moral Worth and Embryos*, ed. Stephen Napier (Dordrecht: Springer, 2011), 268. Earlier, Alvaré observes that "speaking generally, it appears that the widespread participation of women in nonmarital sexual relations is detrimental to women's well being . . . Far more women than men report that they regret casual sexual encounters regret early sexual encounters, or wish they had waited until they were older, or suffer depression after uncommitted sexual intimacy. Additionally, women, more often than men express negative opinions about cohabitation, and report that they understand cohabitation as a precursor to marriage, (Men), more often understand it as another stage of dating. Finally, it is apparent that women take on disproportionate burdens

within the framework of the current mating market, given that they alone become pregnant, they alone undergo abortions, they unduly suffer from post-abortion distress, and they far more often rear children alone than do men, by a ratio of about eight to one . . . abortion, in particular, both structures the current market to pressure single women toward sexual relations, and then immiserates them relative to men, by burdening them disproportionately with the consequences of these relations" (Alvaré, "Abortion, Sexual Markets and the Law," 263–4).

61 A recent study by a UK abortion provider found that two thirds of women having abortions were using contraception at the time when they became pregnant. The Chief Executive commented that "Ultimately women cannot control their fertility through contraception alone, and need accessible abortion services as a back-up for when their contraception lets them down" (British Pregnancy Advisory Service Press Release: "Women trying hard to avoid unwanted pregnancy, research shows", 4 February 2014, at http://www.bpas.org/bpasknowledge.php?year=2014&npage=0&page=81&news=624). Note also that some standard forms of 'contraception' work, or can work, post-fertilization, raising the question whether couples should not space their children in alternative ways that do not risk harm to their embryos (see note 65 of Chapter 3).

62 For example, a recent Spanish study in the journal *Contraception* observed that "It is interesting and paradoxical that the large increase in elective abortions was associated with (a) a remarkable increase in the number of women who used contraceptive methods (30%) and (b) improvements in the education level during both the study periods" (José Luis Dueñas, Iñaki Lete, Rafael Bermejo et al., "Trends in the Use of Contraceptive Methods and Voluntary Interruption of Pregnancy in the Spanish Population during 1997–2007", *Contraception* 83 (2011): 82–87).

63 For an extended argument for this view, see Alexander Pruss's *One Body*, especially chapter 6. See also Watt, *Fertility and Gender*, especially the chapters by Alexander Pruss and Anthony McCarthy.

64 "As a union as 'one organism,' an act of sexual intercourse by itself falls short in regard to the temporal extension that organisms have. If romantic love's union consisted in a single act of intercourse, that would be disappointing. The couple seeks to be 'one flesh' as truly as is possible for them, but biologically the aspect of duration that organisms have is lacking . . . However, human persons can extend their actions over time through undertaking a commitment. In a *commitment* to a lasting relationship, a couple can extend the biologically momentary nature of the union in intercourse. If they do so, then the union of the couple as one organism involves both of them on the biological level, which yields the common physical striving of the organs of generation, and on the personal level, which commits them to a relationship of the kind of love of which sexual intercourse is the consummation. The temporally extended biological and personal relationship is then a whole, in which the commitment temporally extends the union of intercourse, which intercourse makes the union into a union as one flesh" (Pruss, *One Body*, 164–5).

65 Note that marital love or 'wishing well' need not be romantic love in any strong sense: mere good will and commitment will be enough to avoid harmful instrumentalisation in this area. See Pruss, *One Body* (including p. 258 on arranged marriages).

66 See note 11 of this chapter. Of course, for some couples, fertility will be permanently 'obstructed' in a way they never chose—which does not mean they cannot fully unite sexually, even if this will never cause conception.

67   Dr. Naomi Bloomfield, an obstetrician who is herself the mother of twins, comments thus on twin reduction:

"I couldn't have imagined reducing twins for nonmedical reasons . . . but I had an amnio and would have had an abortion if I found out that one of the babies had an anomaly, even if it wasn't life-threatening. I didn't want to raise a handicapped child. Some people would call that selfish, but I wouldn't. Parents who abort for an anomaly just don't want that life for themselves, and it's their prerogative to fashion their lives how they want. Is terminating two to one really any different morally?" (Padawer, "The Two-Minus-One Pregnancy").

Clearly, there is a whole connected mindset at work here on Dr. Bloomfield's part, taking in not only prenatal 'quality control' and abortion but also, one assumes, IVF and contraception. To say that IVF particularly lends itself to controlling, consumerist attitudes to children is not to deny that such attitudes may also be present with natural pregnancies where the 'setting' in terms of attitudes to sex and fertility will, again, be important.

68   Erika Bachiochi, "Embodied Equality: Debunking Equal Protection Arguments for Abortion Rights", *Harvard Journal of Law & Public Policy* 34.3 (2011), 946.

69   A view of the sperm as an intrusion is sadly all too accurate socially in cases of rape, as opposed to genuine intercourse between a couple. Here we are outside the context of 'contraception' strictly speaking: the specific moral issues raised by contraception apply only to those who are choosing both the intercourse and the prevention of conception. On the question of preventing conception after rape in a way that does not seriously risk, by acting post-fertilization, the life of any embryo who may still be conceived, see Thomas V. Berg, Marie T. Hilliard, and Mark F. Stegman, "Emergency Contraceptives and Catholic Health Care: A New Look at the Science and the Moral Question", *Westchester Institute for Ethics and the Human Person White Paper Series* 2.1 (2011). For a more restrictive approach incorporating new evidence on post-ovulation effects of 'Plan B' in particular, see Rebecca Peck and Juan R. Velez, "The Postovulatory Mechanism of Action of Plan B", *National Catholic Bioethics Quarterly* 13.4 (2013): 677–716 (see also responses in later issues of the journal).

70   Richards, *The Ethics of Parenthood*, 77. In the context of postnatal 'parenting' where one parent works long hours while the other cares for the child, Alexander Pruss points out that parents should be friends of each other, and that quite generally human beings "do act vicariously through our close friends, in such a way that we can say "*We did it*" (Pruss, *One Body*, 382).

71   Richards, *Ethics of Parenthood*, 77–8.

72   Ibid., 78–9.

73   Nicanor Austriaco, "On the Catholic Vision of Conjugal Love and the Morality of Embryo Transfer", in *Human Embryo Adoption: Biotechnology, Marriage, and the Right to Life*, eds. Thomas V. Berg and Edward J. Furton (Philadelphia and Thornwood, New York: Westchester Institute and National Catholic Bioethics Center, 2006), 118.

74   Pincott, *Do Chocolate Lovers Have Sweeter Babies?*

75   Velleman, "Family History", 370–1.

76   See, for example, Colombetti, who refers to "that first structural dependence, source of all the others, that permits man to be and to exist. We need to think of ourselves as beings that have literally taken flesh in relationship, that are not the fruit of self-projection or self-realization, that are from the beginning beings-with" (Colombetti, "Relazione e de-somatizzazione", 203–4).

On the significance of pregnancy with regard to peace, Donald DeMarco arrestingly comments:

"Our age has lost the symbols of peace which could offer to us its positive and active value. If there is to be an honest and fruitful attempt to achieve peace, the dignity and beauty of the mother-with-child must be reinstated. . . . To deny the beauty and the eminently human character of that tranquil and orderly reciprocity which flows between the mother and her unborn child is to suppress the most universal, accessible and prodigious symbol of peace man has ever been granted the privilege to perceive." ("Pregnancy: The Peace Movement Without Peer", in Donald De Marco, *Abortion in Perspective* [Cincinnati, Ohio: Hiltz & Hayes, 1974], 100–104).

77   Colombetti, "Relazione e de-somatizzazione", 199.

78   See Maloney: "Yes, women conceive and bear children, and it is sexual intimacy with men that makes this possible. The world . . . must acknowledge the power and beauty of this possibility, and remake itself in the image of this fact.

What would this mean? It would mean a world in that every human being, male and female, took seriously the power and beauty of sexual communion. It would be a world in which humans agreed that violence solves nothing, and almost always begets more violence. It would be a world which valued and held in highest regard the ability to give birth, and organized itself around the importance of that power. It would be a world in which both fathers and mothers would be expected to rear their children, an activity that would count in their favor in the marketplace. Never would children be treated as either a burden that society tires of paying for, or a hobby that had best be pursued on one's own time. It would be a world in which all human beings, male and female, adult and child, respect the bodily and spiritual integrity of themselves and those around them" (Maloney, "You Say You Want a Revolution?" 40).

Appendix: Pregnancy and Lethal Fetal Anomaly

> I was angry and hurting. I struggled with my feelings towards my baby. I was angry at him for changing my body, angry at him for still being alive two weeks after our diagnosis. I wanted to be done. The guilt set in when I thought about his innocence and contemplated his life, the life that I was being blessed to share a part.[1]

This is the reaction of one woman whose baby was diagnosed prenatally as having a medical condition incompatible with more than brief survival after birth. In such cases, the pregnancy itself, whether or not it will or can go to term, will last for all or almost all the baby's life, and the parents may know this long before birth if the child's condition was accurately diagnosed.

The shattering nature of such a discovery is almost impossible to understand for those who have not experienced it themselves. So painful is the discovery of lethal anomaly that it has often been assumed—even by those normally opposed to abortion—that abortion in this case, at least, is morally justified, as a humane service to the pregnant woman. Women have sometimes been invited, in some times and places, to abort the child the very day of the diagnosis—or at least, to start planning at once for an abortion just as soon as one can be procured. Those women and couples who express an unwillingness to abort may even experience some degree of pressure to reconsider on the part of health professionals who do not share or understand their qualms. [2]

That said, there are signs of change in this regard, as a very different approach to the diagnosis of lethal conditions gains ground. This is the approach known as 'perinatal hospice',[3] which treats such babies much like other children who are terminally ill and whose families need to be supported as they 'accompany' them in their final weeks and days. The increasing acceptance of the perinatal hospice approach in the medical profession, even by those who do not actively support it, may owe something to evidence suggesting that women who continue such pregnancies do better emotionally long-term than those who undergo abortions.[4] Bearing in mind that many parents will themselves regard the fetus as a child, the consistency the perinatal hospice approach offers with society's response to dying children generally will be a strong recommendation. For example, those who oppose non-voluntary euthanasia of children—for example, on the grounds that all human lives have value—may have similar difficulty accepting the abortion of babies who do not have long to live.

In the perinatal hospice approach, parents are supported throughout the remainder of the pregnancy, with all that this involves: communication with friends and family, appreciation of the pregnancy itself as a time to enjoy the baby's living presence, and preparation for birth, which may be accompanied by photographs or videos, a baptism for those who wish it, time for older siblings and other family members to say goodbye to the baby and so on. For all the deep sorrow and pain still involved in the stillbirth or neonatal death of the baby, there is also a sense of peace, and even joy, that parents may report.

Worth noting here is the greater focus on, and valuing of, the pregnancy itself which the situation 'forces', since this may be the only lengthy time the parents will have with their baby. It is often assumed that the only value in pregnancy for the woman comes from the birth of a child who can be raised by her,[5] or at least by other parents. Women and couples whose babies have a lethal anomaly may, however, come to see pregnancy in a very different light. Thus "Monika", one of those quoted in *A Gift of Time*, a book recounting parents' experiences, recalls that:

> What changed was the way I saw my baby during pregnancy. Before, I was just impatient for the moment my baby would be born. The pregnancy didn't count. The diagnosis made me realise that my baby was already important, that I had to enjoy every moment of her life because maybe there would be no 'after'.[6]

So, too, "Jessica" reflects:

> Every day that we were still pregnant felt like a gift. He was happy inside me, he was fine inside me, he was healthy inside me, because he didn't need those things to function well inside me. He didn't need lungs.[7]

A similar thought, though focused more on the sadness of birth, is expressed by "Chris":[8]

> I was worried more about the birth of my daughter than carrying her. What I mean is that as long as she was inside me I knew she was OK. I wanted to stay pregnant with her because then I could keep her. I was so sad about having to say goodbye when she was born.

Here as elsewhere, we should give full weight to the *relational* significance of pregnancy, in spite of (or including) its very real burdens for the woman who is pregnant. As the authors of *A Gift of Time* comment:

Mothers may feel a sense of pride in the power of their bodies and their capacity to nurture and give birth to another human being.[9]

But above all, the pregnancy is about a *specific* relationship with a particular, albeit dying, baby:

> By giving my son the protection of my body to face the announced death, I was giving him life, all of his life, so that it would be recorded in our family, in all of our history, and in the hearts of each of us. It wasn't a morbid walk but a formidable surge of love.[10]

And finally, from "Jamie" come the following words as she remembers the brief life of her daughter Keiran, words which may serve as a fitting end to this Appendix, and to this book as a whole:

> I loved Keiran from the moment I knew she existed. Nothing changed that when I found out that she would die. If anything, I loved her more. I tried to fit a lifetime of love into nine months. She was always loved, always warm and safe inside me. We should all be so lucky that all we know is love.[11]

NOTES

1 Karla, in Kuebelbeck and Davis, *A Gift of Time*, 66.
2 See, for example, the experience of "JoAnne", whose baby was diagnosed as having the lethal condition skeletal dysplasia:
   "We told my doctor that we would not terminate the pregnancy, and he insisted that I speak to a counselor. He gave me a phone number, which I called. I figured the more people I talked to and the more information I gathered, the better prepared I would be. I called the number and began to tell my story to a counselor named Patty. I had no idea that Patty was a counselor for an abortion clinic. After hearing my story, she explained to me that, because I was already twenty-one-weeks pregnant, I had to make an appointment quickly—I only had up to twenty-four weeks to terminate. She then explained that because I was so far along, they would have to do a procedure in which the baby would not be "intact" after removal. I cannot begin to explain the feelings that I had at that moment. It was a combination of sheer horror and complete peace—horror at the thought of killing my baby and peace at the knowledge that my decision to keep the baby was confirmed. We would hold him and kiss him and hug him for as long as God would allow us.
   My husband and I felt very strongly about our decision. We felt that we had signed on to be parents to this baby right from the beginning, and if being his parents meant that our only job was to see him through his short life and make sure that he went with peace, dignity and love, then we have done our job as parents" (Monica Rafie and Tracy Winsor, "Hope after Poor Prenatal Diagnosis", *Ethics and Medics* 36.10 [October 2011]: 1–2).

3　See the website www.perinatalhospice.org

4　Kuebelbeck and Davis, *Gift of Time*, 37.

5　Thus Anca Gheaus claims that "Pregnancy often involves specific benefits as well as costs. However, the benefits and joys of pregnancy do not cancel out the costs, and do not turn pregnancy into an intrinsically desirable experience . . . Other benefits of pregnancy, such as the joyous anticipation of a baby, are only valuable given the assumption that one carries a baby one will keep and raise" (Gheaus, "The Right to Parent One's Biological Baby," 17).

6　*Gift of Time*, 344

7　Ibid., 130–31.

8　Ibid., 71.

9　Ibid., 368.

10　Ibid., 343.

11　Ibid., 364.

Bibliography

Alvaré, Helen. "Abortion, Sexual Markets and the Law." In *Persons, Moral Worth and Embryos,* edited by Stephen Napier, 255–279. Dordrecht: Springer, 2011.

Anonymous. "Making the Best of Bed Rest", http://www.parentingweekly.com/pregnancy/pregnancy-complications/making-the-best-of-bedrest_2.htm.

Anonymous. "An IVF Doctor has a Change of heart." *MercatorNet*, April 19, 2012, http://www.mercatornet.com/articles/view/charge_of_heart.

Anscombe Bioethics Centre. *Clones and Three-Parent Babies: The Ethics of Mitochondrial Replacement.* http://www.bioethics.org.uk/images/user/MitochondrialReplacementBriefing14November2012.

Austriaco, Nicanor. "On the Catholic Vision of Conjugal Love and the Morality of Embryo Transfer." In *Human Embryo Adoption: Biotechnology, Marriage, and the Right to Life,* edited by Thomas V. Berg and Edward J. Furton, 115–134. Philadelphia and Thornwood, New York: Westchester Institute and National Catholic Bioethics Center, 2006.

Austriaco, Nicanor. "Resolving Crisis Pregnancies: Acting on the Mother versus Acting on the Fetal Child." *National Catholic Bioethics Quarterly* 15.2 (2015): 207–8.

Bachiochi, Erika. "Embodied Equality: Debunking Equal Protection Arguments for Abortion Rights." *Harvard Journal of Law & Public Policy* 34.3 (2011): 889–950.

Baker, Lynne Rudder. "When Does a Person Begin?" *Social Policy and Philosophy* 22.2 (2005): 25–48.

Beckwith, Francis J. *Defending Life: A Moral and Legal Case Against Abortion Choice.* Cambridge: Cambridge University Press, 2007.

Beeson, D.R., Jennings, P.K., and Kramer, W. "Offspring Searching for Their Sperm Donors: How Family Type Shapes the Process." *Human Reproduction* 26.9 (2011): 2415–24.

Bellieni, Carlo V., and Buonocore, Giuseppe. "Abortion and Subsequent Mental Health: Review of the Literature." *Psychiatry and Clinical Neurosciences* 67.5 (2013): 301–310.

Ber, Rosalie. "Ethical Issues in Gestational Surrogacy." *Theoretical Medicine* 21 (2000): 153–169.

Berg, T.V., and Furton, E.J. eds. *Human Embryo Adoption: Biotechnology, Marriage, and the Right to Life.* Philadelphia and Thornwood: National Catholic Bioethics Center and Westchester Institute for Ethics and the Human Person, 2006.

Berg, Thomas V., Hilliard, Marie T., and Stegman, Mark F. "Emergency Contraceptives and Catholic Health Care: A New Look at the Science and the Moral Question." *Westchester Institute for Ethics and the Human Person White Paper Series* 2.1 (2011): 1-30

Boonin, David. *A Defense of Abortion*. New York: Cambridge University Press, 2003.

Brake, Elizabeth. "Fatherhood and Child Support: Do Men Have a Right to Choose?" *Journal of Applied Philosophy* 22.1 (2005): 55–70.

Brakman, Sarah-Vaughan, and Weaver, Darlene Fozard eds. *The Ethics of Embryo Adoption and the Catholic Tradition*. Villanova, PA: Springer, 2007.

Bringman, Jay J., and Shabanowitz, Robert B. "The Placenta as an Organ of the Fetus." *National Catholic Bioethics Quarterly* 15 (2015): 31–37.

British Pregnancy Advisory Service Press Release: "Women Trying Hard to Avoid Unwanted Pregnancy, Research Shows", 4 February 2014, at http://www.bpas.org/bpasknowledge.php?year=2014&npage=0&page=81&news=624.

Brock, Stephen. *Action & Conduct: Thomas Aquinas and the Theory of Action*. Edinburgh: T&T Clark, 1998.

Brown, Brandon P., and Eberl, Jason T. "Ethical Considerations in Defense of Embryo Adoption." In *The Ethics of Embryo Adoption and the Catholic Tradition*, edited by Sarah-Vaughan Brakman and Darlene Fozard Weaver, 103–118. Villanova, PA: Springer, 2007.

Bryan, Elizabeth. "Loss in Higher Multipregnancy and Multifetal Pregnancy Reduction." *Twin Research* 5 (2002): 169–74.

Cataldo, Peter J., and Goodwin, T. Murphy. "Early Induction of Labor." In *Catholic Health Care Ethics: A Manual for Practitioners*, second edition, edited by Edward J.Furton with Peter J.Cataldo and Albert S. Moraczewski, 111–118. Philadelphia, PA: National Catholic Bioethics Center, 2009.

Cataldo, Peter J., Cusick, William, Gremmels, Becket *et al.* "Deplantation of the Placenta in Maternal-Fetal Vital Conflicts." *National Catholic Bioethics Quarterly* 15.2 (2015): 341–250.

Centre for Social Justice. *Response: Child Poverty and Improving Life Chances*, 18 February, 2011. http://www.centreforsocialjustice.org.uk/publications/response-child-poverty-and-improving-life-chances.

Clark, Katrina. "My Father Was an Anonymous Sperm Donor." *Washington Post*, December 7, 2006, http://www.washingtonpost.com/wp-dyn/content/article/2006/12/15/AR2006121501820.html.

Coleman, P.K. "Abortion and Mental Health: Quantitative Synthesis and Analysis of Research Published 1995–2009." *British Journal of Psychiatry* 199 (2011): 180–186.

Colombetti, Elena. "Relazione e de-somatizzazione: Per un approccio relazionale al tema della generazione extracorporea." *Medicina e Morale* 62 (2012): 191–208.

Condic, Maureen. "When Does Human Life Begin? A Scientific Perspective." Westchester Institute White Paper 1.1 (2008):1-18

Coope, Christopher. *Worth and Welfare in the Controversy over Abortion*. London: Palgrave Macmillan, 2006.

DeGrazia, David. "Moral Status, Human Identity, and Early Embryos: A Critique of the President's Approach." *Journal of Law, Medicine and Ethics* 34.1 (2006): 49–57.

de Lacey, Sheryl. "Parent identity and 'Virtual' Children: Why Patients Discard Rather Than Donate Unused Embryos." *Human Reproduction* 20.6 (2005): 1661–1669.

Dellapenna, Joseph W. *Dispelling the Myths of Abortion History*. Durham, NC: Carolina Academic Press, 2006.

DeMarco, Donald. *Abortion in Perspective*. Cincinnati, Ohio: Hiltz & Hayes, 1974.

Denis, Lara. "A Kantian Approach to Abortion." *Philosophy and Phenomenological Research* 76.1 (2008): 117–137.

Denyer, Nicholas. "Is Anything Absolutely Wrong?" In *Human Lives: Critical Essays on Consequentialist Bioethics,* edited by David S. Oderberg and Jacqueline A.Laing, 39–57. London: Palgrave Macmillan, 1997.

DiCamillo, John A., and Edward J. Furton. "Early Induction and Double Effect." *National Catholic Bioethics Quarterly* 15.2 (2015): 251–261.

Diprose, Rosalyn. *The Bodies of Women.* London: Routledge, 1994.

Draper, E.S., Alfirevic, Z. *et al.* "An investigation into the reporting and management of late terminations of pregnancy (between 22 +0 and 26 +6 weeks of gestation) within NHS Hospitals in England in 2006: the EPICure preterm cohort study." *BJOG: An International Journal of Obstetrics and Gynaecology* 119 (2012), published online 7 March 2012, DOI: 10.1111/j.1471–0528.2012.03285.x.

Dreger, Alice Domurat. "The Limits of Individuality: Ritual and Sacrifice in the Lives and Medical Treatment of Conjoined Twins." *Stud. Hist. Phil. Biol. & Biomed. Sci.* 29.1 (1998): 1–29.

Dueñas, José Luis, Lete, Iñaki, Bermejo, Rafael *et al.* "Trends in the use of contraceptive methods and voluntary interruption of pregnancy in the Spanish population during 1997–2007." *Contraception* 83 (2011): 82–87.

Dworkin, Ronald. *Life's Dominion: An Argument About Abortion, Euthanasia, and Individual Freedom.* London: Harper Collins, 1993.

Eberl, Jason T. "Metaphysical and Moral Status of Cryopreserved Embryos." *Linacre Quarterly* 79.3 (2012): 304–315.

Ehrich, Kathryn, Williams, Clare, and Farsides, Bobbie. "The embryo as moral work object: PGD/IVF staff views and experiences." *Sociology of Health and Illness* 30.5 (2008): 772–787.

Fabre, Cecile. *Whose Body Is It Anyway?* Oxford: Clarendon, 2006.

Farmer, Ann. *By Their Fruits: Eugenics, Population Control, and the Abortion Campaign.* Washington: Catholic University of America Press, 2008.

Feinstein, Sharon. "Celibate Woman Plans to Have 3 Babies." *Mirror,* July 10, 2005, http://www.people.co.uk/archive/other/2005/07/10/celibate-woman-plans-to-have-3-babies-102039–15719946/.

Ferguson, D.M., Horwood, L.J., and Boden, J.M. "Abortion and mental health disorders: Evidence from a 30 year longitudinal study." *British Journal of Psychiatry* 193 (2008): 444–51.

Ferguson, David M., Horwood, L. John, and Boden, Joseph M. "Does abortion reduce the mental health risks of unwanted or unintended pregnancy? A reappraisal of the evidence." *Australian and New Zealand Journal of Psychiatry,* DOI: 10.1177/0004867413484597, published online 3 April 2013.

Finnis, John. "The Rights and Wrongs of Abortion: A Reply to Judith Thomson." *Philosophy and Public Affairs* 2.2 (1973): 117–145.

Finnis, John, Grisez, Germain, and Boyle, Joseph. ""Direct" and "Indirect": A reply to critics of our action theory." *Thomist* 65.1 (2001): 1–44.

Flannery, Kevin. "Vital Conflicts and the Catholic Magisterial Tradition." *National Catholic Bioethics Quarterly* 11.4 (2011): 691–704.

Fleming, Patrick M. Review of *The Dignity of Human Procreation and Reproductive Technologies: Anthropological and Ethical Aspects. Humanum* (Summer 2012), http://www.humanumreview.com/articles/view/pontifical-academy-for-life-dignity-of-human-procreation.

Garcia, J.L.A. "Intentions in Medical Ethics." In *Human Lives: Critical Essays on Consequentialist Bioethics,* edited by David Oderberg and Jacqueline Laing, 161–181. London: Macmillan, 1997.

Garcia, J.L.A. "The Doubling Undone? Double Effect in Recent Medical Ethics." *Philosophical Papers* 36.2 (2007): 245–270.

Garcia, J.L.A. "The Primacy of the Virtuous." *Philosophia* 20 (1990): 69–91.

Garcia, J.L.A. "The Virtues of the Natural Moral Law." In *Natural Law in Contemporary Society*, edited by Holger Zaborowski, 99–140. Washington: Catholic University of America Press, 2010.

Garcia, Laura. "Authentic Freedom and Equality in Difference". In *Women, Sex, and the Church*, edited by Erika Bachiochi, 15–33. Boston: Pauline Books & Media, 2010.

Geach, Mary. "Motherhood, IVF and Sexual Ethics." In *Fertility and Gender*, edited by Helen Watt, 169–183. Oxford: Anscombe Bioethics Centre, 2011.

Gentry, Heather. "No Kids For Me, Thanks: I Don't Enjoy Alien-Parasites." *Slate*, June 12, 2012.

George, Robert P., and Christopher Tollefsen. *Embryo: A Defense of Human Life*. New York: Doubleday, 2008.

Gheaus, Anca. "The Right to Parent One's Biological Baby." *Journal of Political Philosophy* 20.4 (2012): 432–455.

Giubilini, Alberto, and Francesca Minerva. "After-birth abortion: why should the baby live?" *Journal of Medical Ethics* 39 (2013): 261–263.

Gómez-Lobo, Alfonso. "Individuality and Human Beginnings: A Reply to David DeGrazia." *Journal of Law, Medicine and Ethics* 35.3 (2007): 457–462.

Grisez, Germain. "Should a woman try to bear her dead sister's frozen embryo?" In Germain Grisez, *The Way of the Lord Jesus, Vol.3: Difficult Moral Questions*, 239–244. Quincy, IL: Franciscan Press, 1997.

Grisez, Germain, Boyle, Joseph, and Finnis, John. "Practical principles, moral truth, and ultimate ends." *American Journal of Jurisprudence* 32 (1987): 99–151.

Hardy, Frances. "Sarah Fletcher has a vocation: she makes babies for other women." *Daily Mail*, March 23, 1996, http://www.highbeam.com/doc/1G1–111418642.html.

Harris, John. *Wonderwoman and Superman: The Ethics of Human Biotechnology*. Oxford: Oxford University Press, 1992.

Harris, Lisa H. "Second Trimester Abortion Provision: Breaking the Silence and Changing the Discourse." *Reproductive Health Matters* 16.31 (2008), Supplement: 74–81.

Hayden, Mary. "The 'Feminism' of Aquinas' Natural Law: Relationships, Love and New Life." In *Abortion: A New Generation of Catholic Responses,* edited by Stephen J. Heaney, 237–242. Braintree, Mass: The Pope John Center, 1992.

Hervé, Fernandez, Capmas, Perrine *et al.* "Fertility after ectopic pregnancy: the DEMETER randomized trial." *Human Reproduction* 28 (2013): 1247–1253.

Holmes, M.M., Resnick, H.S., Kilpatrick, D.G., Best, C.L. "Rape-related pregnancy: estimates and descriptive characteristics from a national sample of women." *American Journal of Obstetrics and Gynecology* 175.2 (1996): 320–4; discussion 324–5.

Hopkins, Patrick D. "Can Technology Fix the Abortion Problem? Ectogenesis and the Real Issues of Abortion." *International Journal of Applied Philosophy* 22.2 (2008): 311–326.

Hursthouse, Rosalind. *Beginning Lives*. Oxford: Blackwell, 1987.

Jadva, V., Freeman, T., Kramer, W., and Golombok, S. "The experiences of adolescents and adults conceived by sperm donation: comparisons by age of disclosure and family type." *Human Reproduction* 24.8 (2009): 1909–19.

Joyce, Mary Rosera. "Are Women Controlling Their Own Minds? The Power of Puritan and Playboy Mentalities." In *Abortion: A New Generation of Catholic Responses*, edited by Stephen J. Heaney, 219–236. Braintree, Mass: The Pope John Center, 1992.

Joyce, Robert. "The Human Zygote Is A Person." In *Abortion: A New Generation of Catholic Responses*, edited by Stephen J. Heaney, 29–42. Braintree, M.A.: The Pope John Center, 1992.

Kaczor, Christopher. *The Ethics of Abortion: Women's Rights, Human Life, and the Question of Justice.* Routledge: New York and London, 2011.

Kaczor, Christopher. "The Ethics of Ectopic Pregnancy: A Critical Reconsideration of Salpingostomy and Methotrexate." *Linacre Quarterly* 76.3 (2009): 265–282.

Kaczor, Christopher. Notes and Abstracts. *National Catholic Bioethics Quarterly* 11 (2011): 579–585.

Kaebnick, Gregory E. "The Natural Father: Genetic Paternity Testing, Marriage, and Fatherhood." *Cambridge Quarterly of Healthcare Ethics* 13 (2004): 49–60.

Kamm, Frances. "Embryonic Stem Cell Research: A Moral Defense." *Boston Review*, October/November 2002, http://bostonreview.net/BR27.5/kamm.html, reprinted in Frances Kamm,

Kamm, Frances. *Bioethical Prescriptions to Create, End, Choose, and Improve Lives.* Oxford and New York: Oxford University Press, 2013.

Keown, John. *Abortion, Doctors and the Law.* Cambridge: Cambridge University Press, 1988.

Kuebelbeck, Amy, and Deborah L. Davis. *A Gift of Time: Continuing Your Pregnancy when your Baby's Life Is Expected to Be Brief.* Baltimore: The Johns Hopkins University Press, 2011.

Lee, Patrick. *Abortion and Unborn Human Life*, second edition. Washington: Catholic University of America Press, 2010.

Lee, Patrick. "Substantial Identity, Rational Nature, and the Right to Life." In *Bioethics with Liberty and Justice*, edited by Christopher Tollefsen, 23–40. Dordrecht: Springer, 2011.

Liao, Matthew. "Time-Relative Interests and Abortion." *Journal of Moral Philosophy* 4 (2007): 242–256.

Lillehammer, Hallvard. "Who cares where you come from? Cultivating virtues of indifference". In *Relatedness in Assisted Reproduction: Families, Origins and Identities*, edited by Tabitha Freeman, Susanna Graham, Fatemeh Ebtehaj, Martin Richards, 97–112. Cambridge: Cambridge University Press, 2014.

Lintott, Sheila. "The Sublimity of Gestating and Giving Birth: Toward a Feminist Conception of the Sublime." In *Philosophical Inquiries into Pregnancy, Childbirth, and Mothering*, edited by Sheila Lintott and Maureen Sander-Staudt, 237–250. New York: Routledge, 2012.

Little, Margaret Olivia. "Abortion, Intimacy, and the Duty to Gestate." *Ethical Theory and Moral Practice* 2 (1999): 295–312.

Long, Stephen A. *The Teleological Grammar of the Moral Act.* Ave Maria, Florida: Sapientia Press, 2007.

McCarthy, Anthony. "Marriage and Meaning." In *Fertility and Gender: Issues in Reproductive and Sexual Ethics*, edited by Helen Watt, 45–69. Oxford: Anscombe Bioethics Centre, 2011.

McCarthy, Anthony. "Unintended Morally Determinative Aspects (UMDAs): Moral Absolutes, Moral Acts and Physical Features in Reproductive and Sexual Ethics." *Studia Philosophiae Christianae* 51.2 (2015): 143–158.

McCarthy, Anthony. *Ethical Sex: Sexual Choices and their Nature and Meaning.* Forthcoming.

McCombs, Phil. "Remembering Thomas." *The American Feminist* 5.1 (1998): 11, http://www.feministsforlife.org/remembering-thomas/.

McMahan, Jeff. *The Ethics of Killing: Problems at the Margins of Life.* New York: Oxford University Press, 2002.

McWhinnie, Alexina. "Gamete Donation and Anonymity: Should Offspring from Donated Gametes Continue to be Denied Knowledge of Their Origins and Antecedents?" *Human Reproduction* 16 (2001): 807–817.

McWhinnie, Alexina, Rose, Joanna, Whipp, Christine, and Jamieson, Louise. *Who Am I: Experiences of Donor Conception*. Leamington Spa: Idreos Education Trust, 2006.

Mahlstedt, Patricia P., LaBounty, Kathleen, and Kennedy, William Thomas. "The Views of Adult Offspring of Sperm Donation: Essential Feedback for the Development of Ethical Guidelines with the Practice of Assisted Reproductive Technology in the United States." *Fertility and Sterility* 93.7 (2010): 2236–2246.

Maloney, Anne M. "Cassandra's Fate: Why Feminists Ought to Be Pro-Life." In *Abortion: A New Generation of Catholic Responses*, edited by Stephen J. Heaney, 209–217. Braintree, MA: The Pope John Center, 1992.

Maloney, Anne. "You Say You Want a Revolution? Pro-Life Philosophy and Feminism." *Life and Learning 5* (1995): 36–37.

Manninen, Bertha. "Pleading Men and Virtuous Women: Considering the Role of the Father in the Abortion Debate." *International Journal of Applied Philosophy* 21.1 (2007): 1–24.

Manninen, Bertha Alvarez. "Rethinking Roe V. Wade: Defending the Abortion Right in the Face of Contemporary Opposition." *American Journal of Bioethics* 10.12 (2010): 33–46.

Manninen, Bertha Alvarez. "The Pro-Choice Pro-Lifer: Battling the False Dichotomy." In *Coming to Life: Philosophies of Pregnancy, Childbirth, and Mothering*, edited by Sarah LaChance Adams and Caroline R. Lundquist, 171–192. New York: Fordham University Press, 2013.

Manning, Wendy D., and Kathleen A. Lamb. "Adolescent Well-Being in Cohabiting, Married, & Single Parent Families." *Journal of Marriage and Family* 65 (2003): 876–893.

Marquardt, Elizabeth, Glenn, Norval D., and Clark, Karen. *My Daddy's Name Is Donor: A New Study of Young Adults Conceived through Sperm Donation*. New York: Commission on Parenthood's Future, 2010.

Mattingly, Susan S. "The Maternal-Fetal Dyad: Exploring the Two-Patient Obstetric Model." *Hastings Center Report* (January–February 1992): 16–17.

Moore, Kristin Anderson, Jekielek, Susan M., and Emig, Carol. *Marriage from a Child's Perspective: How Does Family Structure Affect Children and What Can We Do about It?* Child Trends Research Brief, June 2002.

Mullin, Amy. *Reconceiving Pregnancy and Childcare: Ethics, Experience, and Reproductive Labour*. New York: Cambridge University Press, 2005.

Munday, Liza. "Souls on Ice: America's Embryo Glut and the Wasted Promise of Stem Cell Research." *Mother Jones Magazine*, July-August, 2006, http://motherjones.com/politics/2006/07/souls-ice-americas-embryo-glut-and-wasted-promise-stem-cell-research.

Mundy, Liza. "Too Much to Carry?" *Washington Post*, May 20, 2007, http://www.washingtonpost.com/wpdyn/content/article/2007/05/15/AR2007051501730.html.

Nelson, Hilda Lindemann. "The Architect and the Bee: Some Reflections on Postmortem Pregnancy." *Bioethics* 8.3 (1994): 247–267.

Oderberg, David S. "Modal Properties, Moral Status, and Identity". *Philosophy and Public Affairs* 26 (1997): 259–298.

Oderberg, David S., and Jacqueline A. Laing, eds. *Human Lives: Critical Essays on Consequentialist Bioethics*. London: Palgrave Macmillan, 1997.

Oehlschlaeger, Fritz. *Procreative Ethics: Philosophical and Christian Approaches to Questions at the Beginning of Life*. Eugene, OR: Cascade Books, 2010.

Olson, Eric T. *The Human Animal: Personal Identity without Psychology*. New York: Oxford University Press, 1997.

Ozolins, John. "Surrogacy: Exploitation or Violation of Intimacy?", http://www.bu.edu/wcp/Papers/OApp/OAppOzol.htm, 3–5.

Padawer, Ruth. "The Two-Minus-One Pregnancy." *New York Times*, August 10, 2011, http://www.nytimes.com/2011/08/14/magazine/the-two-minus-one-pregnancy.html?pagewanted=all.

Parfit, Derek. *Reasons and Persons*. Oxford: Clarendon, 1984.

Parke, Mary. *Are Married Parents Really Better for Children? What Research Says About the Effects of Family Structure on Child Well-Being*. Washington, DC: Center for Law and Social Policy, 2003.

Paske, Gerald H. "Sperm-napping and the Right Not to Have a Child." *Australasian Journal of Philosophy* 6.1 (1987): 98–103.

Peck, Rebecca, and Juan R. Velez. "The Postovulatory Mechanism of Action of Plan B." *National Catholic Bioethics Quarterly* 13.4 (2013): 677–716.

Piering, Julie. "The Pregnant Body as a Public Body: An Occasion for Community Care, Instrumental Coercion, and a Singular Collectivity." In *Philosophical Inquiries into Pregnancy, Childbirth, and Mothering*, edited by Sheila Lintott and Maureen Sander-Staudt, 178–190. New York: Routledge, 2012.

Pincott, Jena. *Do Chocolate Lovers Have Sweeter Babies?* New York: Free Press, 2011.

Porter, Lindsey. "Adoption Is Not Abortion-Lite." *Journal of Applied Philosophy* 29.1 (2012): 63–78.

Prewitt, Shauna R. "Giving Birth to a "Rapist's Child": A Discussion and Analysis of the Limited Legal Protections Afforded to Women Who Become Mothers Through Rape." *Georgetown Law Journal* 98 (2010): 827–862.

Pruss, Alexander. "Maternal Love and Abortion", http://www9.georgetown.edu/faculty/ap85/papers/MaternalLoveandAbortion.html.

Pruss, Alexander. "I Was Once a Fetus: That Is Why Abortion Is Wrong." In *Persons, Moral Worth and Embryos,* edited by Stephen Napier, 19–42. Dordrecht: Springer, 2011.

Pruss, Alexander. *One Body: An Essay on Christian Sexual Ethics*. Notre Dame, IN: Notre Dame Studies in Ethics and Culture, 2012.

Rafie, Monica, and Tracy Winsor. "Hope after Poor Prenatal Diagnosis." *Ethics and Medics* 36.10 (October 2011): 1–2.

Rajczi, Alex. "Abortion, Competing Entitlements, and Parental Responsibility." *Journal of Applied Philosophy* 26 (2009): 379–395.

Rape Crisis Network, Ireland. "What Does RCNI National Data Collection Tell Us about Rape Survivors and Termination of Pregnancy?", http://www.rcni.ie/uploads/RangeOfOutcomesOfSurvivorsOfRapeWhoArePregnantAsAResultOfRape2011.pdf.

Reardon, David C., Makimaa, Julie, and Sobie, Amy, eds. *Victims and Victors: Speaking Out About Their Pregnancies, Abortions, and Children Resulting from Sexual Assault*. Springfield, IL: Acorn Books, 2000.

Reist, Melinda Tankard. *Giving Sorrow Words: Women's Stories of Grief After Abortion*. Sydney: Duffy & Snellgrove, 2000.

Reist, Melinda Tankard. *Defiant Birth: Women Who Resist Medical Eugenics*. Melbourne: Spinifex, 2006.

Reist, Melinda Tankard. "The birth mother not the gestational carrier gave nic and keith a baby", http://melindatankardreist.com/2011/01/the-birth-mother-not-the-gestational-carrier-gave-nic-and-keith-a-baby/.

Rhonheimer, Martin. *Vital Conflicts in Medical Ethics: A Virtue Approach to Craniotomy and Tubal Pregnancies*. Washington, DC: Catholic University of America Press, 2009.

Richards, Norvin. *The Ethics of Parenthood*. Oxford and New York: Oxford University Press, 2010.

Roberts, Helen, and Frances Hardy. "Our 'rent a womb' child from an Indian baby farm", *Daily Mail*, August 31, 2012 (updated September 1, 2012), http://www.

dailymail.co.uk/femail/article-2196538/Our-rent-womb-child-Indian-baby-farm-British-couple-paying-20–000-desperately-poor-single-mother-child.html#ixzz26AEYdVBN.

Rose, Joanna. "Kinship: Are Some More Equal Than Others?" In Alexina McWhinnie, Joanna Rose, Christine Whipp, Louise Jamieson, *Who Am I: Experiences of Donor Conception*, 1–13. Leamington Spa: Idreos Education Trust, 2006.

Ross, Steven L. "Abortion and the Death of the Fetus." *Philosophy & Public Affairs* 11 (1982): 232–224.

Rothman, Barbara Katz. *The Tentative Pregnancy*. New York: Penguin, 1986.

Rothman, Barbara Katz. *Recreating Motherhood: Ideology and Technology in a Patriarchal Society*. New York and London: W.W. Norton & Co., 1989.

Savulescu, Julian. "Future People, Involuntary Medical Treatment in Pregnancy and the Duty of Easy Rescue." *Utilitas* 19 (2007): 1–20.

Scheffler, Samuel. *Consequentialism and Its Critics*. Oxford: Oxford University Press, 1988.

Schueneman, Brooke. "Creating Life, Giving Birth, and Learning to Die." In *Philosophical Inquiries into Pregnancy, Childbirth, and Mothering*, edited by Sheila Lintott and Maureen Sander-Staudt, 165–177. New York: Routledge, 2012.

Sharma, Alok, and Pratap Kumar. "Understanding Implantation Window, a Crucial Phenomenon." *Journal of Human Reproductive Sciences* 5.1 (2012): 1–2.

Shewmon, D. Alan. "Brain Death: Can It Be Resuscitated?" *Hastings Center Report* 39.2 (2009): 18–24.

Singer, Peter. *Practical Ethics*, third edition. New York: Cambridge University Press, 2011.

Smajdor, Anna. "The Moral Imperative for Ectogenesis." *Cambridge Quarterly of Healthcare Ethics* 16 (2007): 336–345.

Smajdor, Anna. "In Defence of Ectogenesis." *Cambridge Quarterly of Healthcare Ethics* 21 (2012): 90–103.

Sommers, Mary Catherine. "Living Together: Burdensome Pregnancy and the Hospitable Self." In *Abortion: A New Generation of Catholic Responses,* edited by Stephen J. Heaney, 243–261. Braintree, MA: The Pope John Center, 1992.

Sparrow, Robert. "Is It "Every Man's Right to Have Babies If He Wants Them"? Male Pregnancy and the Limits of Reproductive Liberty." *Kennedy Institute of Ethics Journal* 18.3 (2008): 275–299.

Stanford, Joseph B., Parnell, Tracey A., and Boyle, Phil C. "Outcomes from Treatment of Infertility with Natural Procreative Technology in an Irish General Practice." *Journal of the American Board of Family Medicine* 21 (2008): 375–384.

Stith, Richard. "Location and Life: How Stenberg v. Carhart Undercut Roe v. Wade." *William and Mary Journal of Women and the Law* 9.2 (2003): 255–278.

Stumpf, Andrea E. "Redefining Mother: A Legal Matrix for New Reproductive Technologies." *The Yale Law Journal* 96 (1986): 187–208.

Tauer, Carol. "Lives at Stake: How to Respond to a Woman's Refusal of Cesarian Surgery When She Risks Losing Her Child or Her Life." *Health Progress* (Sept 1992): 20–27.

Tham, Elizabeth, Schliep, Karen, and Stanford, Joseph. "Natural Procreative Technology for Infertility and Recurrent Miscarriage: Outcomes in a Canadian Family Practice." *Canadian Family Physician* 58 (May 2012): E267–274.

Thomson, Judith Jarvis. "A Defense of Abortion." *Philosophy & Public Affairs* 1.1 (1971): 47–66.

Tollefsen, Christopher. "Could Human Embryo Transfer Be Intrinsically Immoral?" In *The Ethics of Embryo Adoption and the Catholic Tradition*, edited by Sarah-Vaughan Brakman and Darlene Fozard Weaver, 85–101. Villanova, PA: Springer, 2007.

Tollefsen, Christopher. "Fetal Interests, Fetal Persons, and Human Goods." In *Persons, Moral Worth, and Embryos*, edited by Stephen Napier, 163–184. Dordrecht: Springer, 2011.

Tonti-Filippini, Nicholas. "The Embryo Rescue Debate: Impregnating Women, Ectogenesis, and Restoration from Suspended Animation." In *Human Embryo Adoption: Biotechnology, Marriage, and the Right to Life*, edited by T.V. Berg and E.J. Furton, 69–114. Philadelphia and Thornwood: National Catholic Bioethics Center and Westchester Institute for Ethics and the Human Person, 2006.

Tooley, Michael, Wolf-Devine, Celia, Devine, Philip E., and Jaggar, Alison M. *Abortion: Three Perspectives*. New York and Oxford: Oxford University Press, 2009.

Turner, A.J., and A. Coyle. "What Does It Mean to Be a Donor Offspring? The Identity Experiences of Adults Conceived by Donor Insemination and the Implications for Counselling and Therapy." *Human Reproduction* 15 (2000): 2041–2051.

Valko, Nancy. "The Case against Premature Induction." *Ethics and Medics* 29.5 (May 2004): 1–2.

Van Maren, Jonathon. "Men and Abortion: The Forgotten Accomplices", http://www.unmaskingchoice.ca/blog/2011/09/23/men-and-abortion-forgotten-accomplices.

Velleman, David J. "Family History." *Philosophical Papers* 34.3 (2005): 357–378.

Watt, Helen. "Potential and the Early Human." *Journal of Medical Ethics* 22 (1996): 222–226.

Watt, Helen. "Germ-line Therapy for Mitochondrial Disease: Some Ethical Objections." *Cambridge Quarterly of Healthcare Ethics* 8 (1999): 88–96.

Watt, Helen. *Life and Death in Healthcare Ethics: A Short Introduction*. London: Routledge, 2000.

Watt, Helen. "Beyond Double Effect: Side-effects and Bodily Harm." In *Human Values: New Essays on Ethics and Natural Law*, edited by David Oderberg and Timothy Chappell, 236–251. London: Palgrave MacMillan, 2004.

Watt, Helen. "Becoming Pregnant or Becoming a Mother? Embryo Transfer with and without a Prior Maternal Relationship." In *Human Embryo Adoption: Biotechnology, Marriage, and the Right to Life*, edited by Thomas V. Berg and Edward J. Furton, 55–67. Philadelphia and Thornwood, New York: Westchester Institute and National Catholic Bioethics Center, 2006.

Watt, Helen. "Embryos and Pseudoembryos: Parthenotes, Reprogrammed Oocytes and Headless Clones." *Journal of Medical Ethics* 33.9 (2007): 554–556.

Watt, Helen. "Conjoined Twins: Separation as Lethal Mutilation." In *The Right to Life and the Value of Life,* edited by Jon Yorke, 337–347. Farnham: Ashgate, 2010.

Watt, Helen, ed. *Fertility and Gender: Issues in Reproductive and Sexual Ethics*. Oxford: Anscombe Bioethics Centre, 2011.

Watt, Helen. "Life and Health: A Value in Itself for Human Beings?" *HEC Forum* (2015), DOI 10.1007/s10730-015-9288-2.

Whipp, Christine. "Worrying the Wound: The Hidden Scars of Donor Conception." In *Who Am I: Experiences of Donor Conception*, edited by Alexina McWhinnie, Joanna Rose, Christine Whipp, and Louise Jamieson, 14–29. Leamington Spa: Idreos Education Trust, 2006.

Wolf-Devine, Celia. "Abortion and the 'Feminine Voice.' *Public Affairs Quarterly* 3.3 (1989): 81–97.

Wolf-Devine, Celia. "Postscript to 'Abortion and the 'Feminine Voice'". The Gutting of the Ethics of Care by Carol Gilligan and Nel Noddings", 1993, www.celiawolfdevine.com.

Wolf-Devine, Celia, and Philip E. Devine. "A Communitarian Pro-Life Perspective". In Michael Tooley, Celia Wolf-Devine, Philip E. Devine, Alison M. Jaggar.

Abortion: Three Perspectives, 65–119. New York and Oxford: Oxford University Press, 2009.

Worcester, O.E. "From a Woman Physician: An Open Letter to Dr. W.W. Parker." *Journal of the American Medical Association* 22 (1894): 599, reprinted in "JAMA 100 Years Ago", *JAMA* 271.15 (1994): 1208b.

Wreen, Michael. "Abortion and Pregnancy due to Rape." *Philosophia* 21 (1992): 201–220.

Young, Iris. *Throwing like a Girl and Other Essays in Feminist Philosophy and Social Theory*. Bloomington and Indianapolis: Indiana University Press, 1990.

Index